## WHAT FOLKS ARE SAYING AE
### *FOOD FREEDOM AND FINISH*

Joyce has written a book that is go
of change—change that will last a ~~. ~~ ~~believe that she~~
has discovered the secret to losing weight and keeping it off. God's love
language is obedience and when we do His work, His way, we will succeed.
You are going to love this book as much as I do!
--- Carole Lewis, National Director, First Place 4 Health

*Food, Freedom and Finish Lines* will tell you how to be a big loser!! Here
you will discover the incredible story of how Joyce Ainsworth lost 192
pounds. I love this book because it is so real and practical. Every page
contains helpful tips on living a healthy lifestyle. Read and apply it now to
make the most of the rest of your life.
---Steve Reynolds, Pastor, Capital Baptist Church, Annandale, VA., Author
of *Bod4God* and *Get Off The Couch*

Joyce Ainsworth's journey to wellness began in a moment of despair when
wedding photos revealed what she never wanted to see. She began the race
none of us wants to begin, and her story will inspire and challenge you to find
your finish line too. Her weight loss—over 192 pounds—is only one result
of her new balanced life and freedom. I highly recommend this book.
---Karen Porter, International Speaker and Author of *I'll Bring the Chocolate*

I love it! Very uplifting and a great read, but also extremely motivating. I
started last night and finished it this morning before lunch. I just couldn't
put this book down. Joyce is for real and she tells it like it is. Excellent read
for anyone, young or old, thick or thin. I am so motivated!
---Jan Duke, Administrative Assistant to the Superintendent of Rankin
County School District.

## FIVE STAR REVIEWS FROM AMAZON

One of the best books I have ever read. Truly life changing, and all the glory
is given to the Lord by the author. An incredible story and I love the way she
relates her journey to running. Look for this book to be a "best seller." Start
your life change today—read the book! ---Donna

This book was hard to put down. I cried with my sweet wife because I can see and understand this tough journey in a different light now. In many places I could see myself in this journey as well because we all face some sort of addiction. Thanks for writing this book and being real and transparent. Only by the power of Christ can any of us be set free. Thanks for sharing the truth with others and thanks for allowing me to be part of the "Life Change." We will run the next race together! By His Grace! ---Glenn

I enjoyed this book. It is a life journey of a lady giving Christ first place in her life, I read this book in 3 days but I re-read parts of each day. I also enjoyed the testimonies of the friends that have lost weight learning to give Christ first place.  ----Gwen

Joyce Ainsworth shares some very painful parts of her life in this revealing book, as an inspiration for others to understand that losing weight must begin on the inside. She helps the reader face reality about how they arrived at their current weight. She gives practical-no-bones ideas about the how-to of making lifestyle changes that are doable. She doesn't just tell how she lost over 192 pounds; she makes it visibly possible for the reader to believe that it is also possible for them. Joyce is a motivating speaker who is real and her compassion for others is real. This book hopefully, is just the first of her victory story!  ---June

This is the wonderfully inspiring story of Joyce Ainsworth, who takes the reader through her weight loss journey (192 pounds!). You read about her highs and lows, struggles and victories. And, then you have the courage to start your own race with your sights on the finish line!  ---Sarah

I read this book with laughter and tears, I saw myself through these pages. I recently met Joyce at First Place 4Health Summit; what an amazing lady! I will keep this book as part of my strength resources through my freedom from food journey. Thank you Joyce for being so real and encouraging.  ---Sarah

Finally! I've been "trying" to lose weight for over 30 years! This book finally told me how with no punches pulled. Nothing "warm and fuzzy" about this lady. LOL I weigh less now than I have in 25 years and have run two 1/2 marathons. Thank you Joyce.   ---Dave

Food, Freedom, and Finish Lines!

"Now includes a New Study Guide"

Food, Freedom, and Finish Lines!

How to Lose the Weight and Win Back Your Life

"Now includes a New Study Guide"


By Joyce Ainsworth

Originally published by Bold Vision Books, Friendswood, Texas

Printed in the U.S.A.

ISBN – 13: 978-1499638486
ISBN – 10: 149 9638485

Cover by Jerome Duran.

# Acknowledgments

I am grateful for the love and support of my friends and staff at my home church Crossgates Baptist Church. They have been willing to step out in faith and provide support for the ministry of First Place 4 Health (FP4H). Thank you for allowing my ministry to flourish and grow here in this place!

I am also very thankful for all the friends and members who have come through my classes. You have touched my life in so many special ways and as we have studied, prayed, and grown together, my desire is that you have been inspired to find real life change. You have encouraged me to share my story so that other lives may be changed as well. Thank you.

A special little thanks to my granddaughter Hannah for being my "beach buddy." I pray we never tire of the small things like picking up seashells together. Hugs to my son Daniel for being my partner in that first half marathon; you really did help me make it to the finish line! A special prayer of thanks to Crystal my sweet daughter in love for allowing me to walk the 12K's of Christmas with you. Crystal, you have taught me great lessons in perseverance and endurance.

I am grateful to Teresa Russell, Kathy Nelson, and Keeli O'Cain for being willing to share their stories with readers through this book. My deepest gratitude and appreciation to Donna Conerly for sharing her story, and sharing her running thoughts and perspectives after and before each race, and the many hours of prayer and support for me as I have ventured to capture the true essence of life change through the pages of this book. Donna and Mike, the two of you have been my "running buddies" in more ways than one. Thank you for allowing Jesus to be real in your lives!

Additional thanks to Dr. Kenneth Barraza for his time in answering countless questions for the interview within this book and to my "fitness friends" at The Club Fitness Center for their invaluable help in understanding the importance of exercise, the inside scoop on racing, the right gear, and many other helpful tips they provided during this journey. They really do believe fitness should be fun.

Thank you, Delilah Dirksen, NE Regional Team Leader for FP4H, for helping put together the website resources in this book and Kristie Armstrong for your beautiful gift of photography.

I will be forever grateful to the dedicated staff of First Place 4 Health. Their willingness to follow the Lord's calling through the ministry of FP4H has radically changed my life. Thank you Carole Lewis for being real and transparent; you have inspired me to be the best I can be!

I am deeply indebted to my dear friend Jan Duke and my husband Glenn for their invaluable work of editing this project. A great big "Thank You" for going above and beyond to make this project the best it could be.

I want to especially thank June Chapko for her guidance and help with the new study guide that has been added. It is an honor to work alongside dear ones like June who love the Lord and allow that to be reflected in their work. May the Lord receive all the Glory!

## Dedication

"Call to me and I will answer you, and I will tell you great and mighty things, which you do not know" (Jeremiah 33:3 NASB).

This book is lovingly and affectionately dedicated to my Savior and Friend Jesus who loved me enough to not leave me in the condition I was in. He has truly made real and lasting life change possible.

~~All for His Glory~~

To my beloved husband Glenn who has always loved "both" of me! Words are inadequate to express my love and gratitude for your steadfast love, encouragement, and support through this life-change journey! Thank you for being willing to run the race.

To my children Heather, David, Daniel, Jason, and Brad. My prayer is for each of you to find real life change through the power of Christ!

To all my readers

Change Your Mind! Change Your Body! Change Your Life!

# Table of Contents

# Introduction

# The Finish Line!

*As I make the final turn on the course, I see it—the finish line! Finally! It is just ahead within my view. My body aches and it seems I can feel every bone in my tired feet. I feel the sweat as it drips between my shoulder blades and then trickles down the center of my back. There is a salty film along my arms from perspiration; my clothes stick to my damp skin. My vision is blurred from sweat. No, on second thought, I think tears are leaking from the corners of my eyes. This has been the longest and hardest journey. I am so tired. I look up and once more see the finish line ahead. From somewhere deep inside, I sense an unnatural surge of energy, and my feet become faster and my body, lighter.*

Who could imagine starting a race weighing in at 339 pounds and now coming this close to the finish!

Some call it the battle of the bulge and others, the great cover-up. I call it addiction, a constant obsession with food. It not only hurts our physical bodies but also entangles and strangles our thoughts, emotions, and minds. Only the power of Christ enables us to find true and lasting freedom.

If you have picked up this book, you are either struggling with or have struggled with weight issues, or perhaps you have surrendered to an unhealthy lifestyle. Whether you have a lot of weight to lose or you are struggling with those last few pounds, never truly finding complete victory, take heart. The finish line is just ahead.

If you are like me, you have read countless how-to books on weight loss. I think I have read everything written, and yet I never found real or lasting success until now. True victory is when you stop dieting and make a life change. Real changes can and will sustain you for a lifetime, but more than change, I invite you to freedom - freedom from the bondage of food.

Conquering food addiction is not about depriving yourself. Instead, it is about freedom. Christ came to set us free. And His freedom includes freedom from food addiction.

*I am almost there, and this time I am determined to finish. My goal is just ahead. No more stopping or falling back. No more.* As I run the race, I look to my left and my right and there they are—my friends, the ones I've met along the way.

"I can't make it; go on without me," words from my friend on my left.

I respond, "I am not going to leave you behind; we are going together even if I have to carry you. Now, let's keep going."

My friend on the right encourages, "You can do it." Together we keep pressing on, one foot in front of the other.

As I share my personal struggle with food and my loss of 192 pounds (a whole person), and the principles I've learned, I pray my story will inspire and encourage you. May you find the courage to begin or finish your own race to real and lasting life change. Now is the time to start living in freedom.

My motto is, "Change your mind. Change your body. Change your life."

Faithfully His,
*Joyce*

"Brothers and sisters, I do not consider myself yet to have taken hold of it. But one thing I do: Forgetting what is behind and straining toward what is ahead, I press on toward the goal to win the prize for which God has called me heavenward in Christ Jesus" (Philippians 3:13-14 NIV).

~

## Chapter 1
## Where Are You? ~ Evaluate to Decide

*I never wanted to run a race. In fact, I couldn't run. I weighed 339 pounds and no one should expect me to run. I didn't come from a family of runners. We celebrate with food, and lots of it! But here I am at the starting line. I don't want to run, yet I don't want to continue as I am. So I will run. I will change the cycle of overeating. The sound of the starting gun splits the air. I take the first step.*

I waited with anticipation to receive the pictures of my daughter's wedding. Heather (our only girl of five children) was the most beautiful bride and I couldn't wait to re-live the wedding through the photographer's eye. And my husband, who was and is my hero, would be in the pictures, too. I eagerly waited for the photo package to arrive in the mail.

As I looked through the pictures, I found my sweet daughter just as lovely as I imagined and my husband as handsome as I had expected. I had forgotten I would be in the photos, too. For most of my life, the only pictures I really liked were ones where I was absent. I gazed into the eyes of the woman in those photos and wondered, "Where am I? The woman in my dress could not possibly be me. Or was it? Was that me!

Pictures have a way of telling us the truth about our looks, but they also give us a glimpse into our soul, those deep, hidden places we rarely let others view. Those wedding photos made me realize I was in terrible and deep bondage. The smile on my face covered up a heart and soul crying out for help. It was a silent cry others could not hear, but on that day, the Lord heard. He whispered across my soul, and for the first time in a long time, I not only could see, but I felt the chains of bondage wrapped tightly around me. I knew I was allowing food to strangle the life out of me.

I have been overweight most of my life and have never really known anything else. I came from a large family with many children to feed. I can still hear Mama say, "Clean your plate. There are children starving to death in other countries." Sound familiar?

On the other side of the coin, Mama also hid food from my siblings and me. She knew if she didn't hide it, we would eat all the food at one time. I'm not sure what she expected when there were six kids reaching for the Little Debbie box, which only came around the circle once. We knew if we didn't grab ours then, we would do without. Sharing was not uppermost in the mind of this child. There always seemed to be enough food for all of us, but it was as if we were constantly surrounded by a fear of never having enough to eat.

As a young overweight teenager, I became the butt of many jokes and much ridicule in and out of school because of my size. Kids say, "Sticks and stones may break my bones but words will never hurt me." But the little poem simply isn't true. Hurtful words cut deep and leave scars that sometimes take a lifetime to heal. I found comfort in food instead of friends.

I look back now and see how from a very young age, I began to develop an unhealthy relationship with food.

Food and obesity became what I call the acceptable sin in my family. My whole family was big, so this made it seem normal and unavoidable. We all seemed healthy, but being overweight was accepted in our family. Yet during quiet moments of desperation and despair, I can still hear my soul crying, *there has to be more to life than this.* When everyone around you is overweight, it is much easier to accept and pretend you are okay in this condition. It was easier to live in the pain than it was to endure the discomfort of change.

When I entered high school, I dieted more and more. I also began to eat in hiding, stuffing the pain and anger as I stuffed my face. I thought life was so unfair. Blaming the overeating on my life situation helped relieve the guilt of eating all the wrong foods. If I tried to diet, I felt deprived, so I ate more. This never-ending cycle only made the anger and the weight worse.

Everyone seemed to be proud of me when I lost a few pounds, but no real change took place in my home to reinforce the changes I'd made in my diet. I carried all my extra weight, emotional bondage, anger, and pain from high school into marriage. I kept looking and searching for answers to the battle. Wearing a size 22, I pretended to be content—you know, the old saying, "Fat and Happy." Don't believe it. The saying is a lie we tell ourselves to escape the pain and shame of obesity.

Years went by, and the struggle continued. I tried one diet program after another, always searching for an answer and never seeming to find any true hope. The weight caused other problems in my life—high blood pressure and cholesterol along with other medical conditions, bad knees and feet, a struggling marriage, overweight children, emotional issues, depression, and poor self-esteem.

Through the years, like so many of us do, I tried every diet and weight-loss pill and all the latest programs and fads. I even got hypnotized one time. When I lost some weight, I always seemed to regain what I lost plus a little more. It was easier to eat than change.

I lived in frustration and defeat. I berated myself with negative self-talk over my lack of self-control and will power. But time and time again, food was my comfort and friend.

People say a picture is worth a thousand words. My daughter's wedding pictures and the question, "Where are you?" became the catalyst that ignited a burning desire in my heart for real change. I asked the Lord to free me from the desperate battle.

Until the day I asked God to free me, I wanted freedom without having to fight for it; I wanted the prize without running the race. It's human nature because Adam and Eve passed this mindset on to us from the beginning. So grab your Bible and look with me in Genesis 3:8-9. "They (Adam and Eve) heard the sound of the Lord God walking in the garden in the cool of the day, and the man and his wife hid themselves from the presence of the Lord God among the trees of the garden. Then the Lord God called to the man, and said to him, 'Where are you?'" (NASB).

In all the times I had read these verses, I had never seen the question before. I guess I was too busy trying to figure out how they made those clothes out of fig leaves. I mean, think about it—two humans trying to hide from an all-seeing, all-knowing God with fig leaves is humorous. God knew every detail about them. He knew where they were. He knows everything about us, too. Maybe He asked the question so they would evaluate their situation honestly.

Eve had a battle with food. According to the Bible, she looked, she took, she ate, and she gave. Eve's desire at this point was not to satisfy hunger for physical food but to meet other needs in her life. The enemy convinced her to eat the fruit because she wanted to be like God. Hunger is a natural and normal response because our bodies need nourishment, but we use food to try to fill all the empty places in our life, instead of the one place God intended it to fill - our stomachs.

Physical hunger is the normal response to a legitimate need. We all experience the feelings of hunger, and eating is the natural response to that feeling. From a very young age, we are taught to eat, not because of a physical hunger but based on emotions. We eat when we are happy, when we are sad, when we are stressed, tired, overworked, or need a break. When we want to show someone we love him or her, we reward him or her with food.

At every wedding, there is food; every party has festive foods; and every holiday has a food with special meaning attached to it. When someone is sick, we cook for them, and even when a person dies, we take food to the family. Now don't get me wrong, I like and enjoy food. There is nothing wrong with good food or celebrations or caring for others' needs. What is wrong is how I tried to fill the other needy areas in my life with food.

Giving food a place God never intended produces intense guilt in my heart and mind, so instead of running to God, I hide from God, just as Adam and Eve hid in the garden. Plain and simple, I try to fill the places of greatest need with physical food.

God has given each of us a hunger for genuine intimacy. Our deepest needs for worth, security, and significance can only be met by the Lord. Only God can fill the wounded place and the place of bondage. Only through Him can we be healed and set free. In the garden, God filled the deepest hunger for Adam and Eve when He came looking for them in the evening. He desires to satisfy your deepest hunger, too. God wanted to be with them, and He longs to be with us. His greatest desire is not to be a part of our lives but to be our lives. He wants to be the centerpiece in my life and your life.

Food was created to bring the physical body nourishment. The natural response to physical hunger is to eat, but we have other hungers not related to the physical need for food. When we try to fill or satisfy the other hungers in our lives with physical food, we have responded unnaturally.

We all have hungers deep within where no one can see. My silent hunger showed up in the eyes of an overweight mother in a wedding picture. My eyes cried out for help; I needed healing from a wounded heart and a fake smile. What place silently cries out in you?

Perhaps the silence has been covered up with years of distorted behavior. We put up protective barriers to still the voice of pain – walls of busyness and the noise and complications of life. Deep hunger cannot be completely silenced; it cries out to be heard. What is your compelling desire? To be loved? Cared for? Protected? Considered precious? My deepest desire was wrapped up in that word "precious." I wanted to be precious.

One day I walked down the beach with Hannah Grace, my granddaughter. I love the beach—the sights, sounds, and smells; the sand; the crashing waves; and the critters in the sea, as long as they don't get near me, and oh, yes, the seashells. I can walk for miles and never get tired of the sights and sounds of the ocean. God always teaches me life lessons in those moments by the sea.

Hannah and I picked up shells from the beach that day. Seashells are amazing. I have hundreds in my collection. Each one is different and has some small imperfection, unique from all the others. Some are broken or have pieces missing; some have lost an edge or a corner, and others boast large, gaping holes. All seem to be weather worn. Most were homes to tiny creatures and may have been victims of a predator. On a rare occasion, I find one with no noticeable imperfections at all.

Hannah Grace held each shell up and regardless of its condition, she said, "Granny, let's keep this one; it is very special to me."

Christ feels the same way about each of us; we are special to Him, and His desire is for us to know how precious we are.

I am so moved by the thought of being precious. As the Lord walks down the beach of our lives, He picks us up, regardless of our condition—tattered, torn, broken, with all our imperfections, all shapes and sizes—and He holds us out to His Father and says, "Let's keep this one; this one is so very special to me, so precious."

God has placed a high value on each of us. His desire is for us to walk close to Him so we will never again doubt how precious we are. God asks us the same question He asked Adam and Eve in the garden: "Where are you?" When I saw myself in those wedding photos, I cried out, "Where am I?"

He knew where I was, but it took a wedding picture for me to be honest with myself. Finally! God wanted to free me from the bondage of food, but He wanted much more. He wanted to walk with me down the beach of life, regardless of the storms that might come. He asked me to face truth. Holding those photos and facing myself helped me see the truth. It was as if the Lord said, "How long will you cry out for help before you allow the one and only great Healer to step into the garden of your life?"

Change will not be easy, but it is possible. When we bring our struggles with food, eating, and weight (or any other addiction for that matter) to Him in honest surrender, He begins the journey with us to our Promised Land. God enters our soul, takes our place of greatest vulnerability and weakness, and uses it to satisfy and heal us. And in the profound silence that accompanies His presence, we hear Him say, "Blessed are those who hunger and thirst for righteousness, for they shall be satisfied" (Matthew 5:6 ESV).

The word "satisfied" in this verse means God wants us to be full, sufficient, and entirely complete, lacking nothing. God uses experiences as a catalyst to mold and make us into the person He calls us to be; not perfect, but healthy, whole, and healed. And to think it all started as I gazed into the beautiful green eyes of a stranger in my daughter's wedding picture. I heard the Lord ask, "Where are you, Joyce?" That day was the beginning of my race.

## * Personal Reflection: Acknowledge the Truth

Being honest with myself was the first step in healing. The journey ahead was not going to be easy, but now I could begin. The honest evaluation allowed me to face the truth. I needed to face my condition - physically, mentally, emotionally, and spiritually. I beat myself up for not having enough will power to lose weight on my own. Coming face to face with the Lord and allowing Him to show me that my addiction to food was sin became my turning point. The bondage in my life was so great; without the supernatural help of the Lord, I was doomed.

Freedom whispered my name, and I finally listened. Will you listen, too?

~ Joyce with her family ~

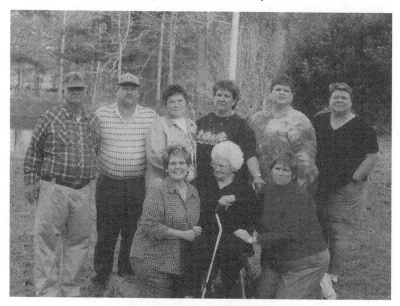

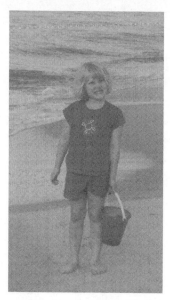

~ Hannah Grace picking up shells ~

~

# Chapter 2
## Attitude Adjustment ~ Start with the Mind

*I hear the warnings from deep within, "You fool. You've tried to run before. You've always failed. Why try now? It's too late for you – already over 300 pounds. There's no hope." I run a few more steps because I really want to finish, but I know I'm sure to fail; again. But another voice whispers into my ear, "Joyce, you are my child, precious and beloved. Run the race. I'll go with you." The voice of my Lord gives me hope, and I swat away those terrible lies of defeat. My mind is clear – I will run.*

As the finish line gets closer, I seem to see more clearly. In the beginning, my mind was so set on failure, everything seemed impossible. As I look back, I smile because now everything seems possible - really. What an attitude change.

How and when did my outlook change? The truth is I always wanted to lose the weight, but it was as if I had another person living in my mind, always setting me up for defeat and failure, instead of success. When I walked into a First Place 4 Health class, the first thing I saw was the scales. I hated the scales. *I cannot get on those scales.* Then I remembered the wedding photos now in residence on my refrigerator. And I remembered the reason I was here.

I got on the scales, and you know what happened next? Nothing. There was no earthquake. The building did not fall down, and no one laughed or made fun of the 339-pound woman on the scales. I felt overwhelming shame, but all I received was love and acceptance. The sweet women around me encouraged me and began to guide me. My physical situation was definitely not where God wanted me to be, and I was not alone.

At that moment, a new thought took root in my mind. All the things I had told myself all those years were lies. I took the next step of my race.

When we alter the way we think, the way we act, the way we feel, and the way we approach life, change will come. First Place 4 Health helps people change in the mental, physical, emotional, and spiritual areas of their lives. I thought I could modify what I ate and change my life alone, but I still longed for the unhealthy choices and could not wait to get off the diet so I could go back to my same old ways. Diets do not work; they never have and never will if real life change is your goal.

Diets do not have lasting results because diets only address the outward behavior. A diet forces the body to make some kind of change, but the mind still desires unhealthy food. Desiring and pursuing unhealthy choices will lead us to slavery. We can become addicted to all sorts of things such as sex, power, alcohol, or possessions. My unhealthy choice happened to be food.

We must change our minds first. When we change our minds, it is much easier for the body to follow where the mind leads.

Learning the lesson of mind change is powerful. Through the FP4H program, I really began to get it.

In the process of trying to change my mind, my body rebelled. I wanted to eat my old standard comfort foods—ice cream and french fries. Each day was a battle. I began losing weight, and then something else happened. My thinking changed about many things, not just food.

One of my First Place leaders said, "We cannot wait until we feel like doing the right things when it comes to food and exercise. Feelings are just emotions." We must not base our decisions on feelings; rather, we must act according to the truth in God's Word. I realized I had approached good health, exercise, and eating properly as negative interruptions instead of as a positive, new lifestyle.

I had to start acting my way into a new approach to feeling. God opened an opportunity for me to become all He wanted me to be. With His help and the FP4H tools, I could do it. But it was up to me to take the next step, see the truth that could set me free, and then act accordingly. My long history of bondage required supernatural strength beyond my control. Guess what? God held my hand, and His strength became my strength. He was there with that first step and has never let go of my hand, and He is with me at the finish line.

With that first step, something amazing happened—a defining moment, a bend in the road, and when I looked up, I saw freedom. That first glimpse ignited a ray of hope in my weary soul. My defining moment came as I was reading from the book of Ephesians. "You were taught, with regard to your former way of life, to put off your old self, which is being corrupted by its deceitful desires; to be made new in the attitude of your minds; and to put on the new self, created to be like God in true righteousness and holiness" (Ephesians 4:22-24 NIV).

This scripture addresses three specific areas of life: the past, the present, and the future. With regard to my former way of life, I was to be done with it. It was as if the Lord said, "Joyce, you have allowed your old self to be in control." It was true. Life had become a vicious cycle for me.

When I experienced overwhelming guilt about my eating habits and my weight gain, I tried to do better. Because I tried to change under my own power, I continually returned to the sin of overeating and unhealthy choices. I was trapped in a sequence of failures. I had no control, yet I was the one in control. I saw my old life in front of me, and God's words pierced my heart. My way of doing things was corrupted by deceitful desires.

The time came to change my mind, but life change required an intentional decision to leave my old life behind. I asked God to bring me out of denial, show me my old self and my motives. I feared the truth would hurt. The path to putting on my new self is the path God created in true righteousness and holiness.

And so, the healing began. Christ forgave me and began to help me shed my old self. The layers came off one by one like peeling an onion.

The first layer had to do with food. I assumed my weight and unhealthy lifestyle (the old me) only hurt me. I was wrong. The underlying poison festered and spread to damage my family and friends, too. I cooked because I loved my family, but the food was unhealthy, and I cooked in unhealthy ways. I was a prisoner to bad choices and I imprisoned them, too, by offering food laden with fat and sugar.

The next layer was not about bad food choices. I needed to peel away layers of bitterness and a critical spirit as well as anger, frustration, and negative self-talk. An unforgiving spirit caused me to hold on to hurts and hang-ups. In my mind, I felt I had never measured up and so the only way to feel better was simply to make sure no one else measured up either. I had failed at so many things in the past, and the only way to cope had been to cover up and pretend. Fake it out; no one would notice! The wounds were deep.

So I latched on to the present tense verb in the next part of the verse from Ephesians, "You need to be made new in the attitude of the mind." The term "made new" is a continual renewing process. My mind and my heart need reprogramming. Life change would not be a one-time fix but a repetitive process.

If I was ever going to be successful, really successful, at the weight-loss journey, I had to spend a lot of time in prayer. So I dropped to my knees and asked God how to accomplish a repetitive and continual renewing of my mind. I admitted my will power was weak.

That prayer was the key to unlocking the door to freedom and power. I did not need more will power but more God power. I had tried in my own strength for way too long and failed miserably. It was time to walk in God's strength.

Daily Bible reading was something I was already doing, but instead of rote reading of my Bible, I began to study it. I didn't worry about how many chapters I could read but concentrated on each verse. I know it sounds crazy, but I was learning to do things in small baby steps. So taking one scripture at a time was doable.

I memorized verses. I repeated them as I walked. I hated walking, but as I planted and replanted God's Word in my mind, walking became fun and enjoyable.

But wait. There's more.

Paul said, "Put on the new self." This final willful decision meant I had to choose to make healthy choices, change the way I ate, where I went, and even who I hung out with. My focus and my goal had to become centered.

The verse gives us a deep look into the heart of our Heavenly Father. He loves us. I was touched by His love. I was encouraged to make new choices and empowered by His strength to be forever changed. My strength and ability to change could only be found in the power of Christ. As I became more dependent upon Christ, I listened and took active steps to adjust my life to become all God called me to be.

When we depend on God, He becomes life. Being healthy and living a healthy lifestyle is a process, and it was as if I had just begun life. Now the race had really begun.

Although I had a new mindset, I did not automatically do all the right things, say all the right things, and think and act the right way. However, I knew if I continued to trust God to change me, He would. Being overweight is a problem of the flesh with a spiritual solution. My problem was not really about the numbers on my scale or what clothing size I wore. It was about the battle raging in my mind. It was about who was in control.

All those years I knew how to lose weight, but what I had been missing was the "want to." Yes, the body wanted to, but the old mind never did.

God taught me little by little. As God controlled my mind, I saw results. The leaders in my group encouraged me to set small achievable goals. My first goal was to weigh less than 300 pounds.

I dropped from 339 pounds to 299 pounds.

As I reached that first mile marker, I knew God was teaching me to have a new mindset. The weight loss and new mindset helped me realize I needed to develop a long-term plan, one that challenged me mentally and physically. My old plan had not pursued a healthy lifestyle. The definition of the word "pursue" is "to follow close upon (someone or something) in a persistent way." A new pursuit meant action, and the idea brought on a wave of fear. I had failed so many times in the past. I had lost weight, only to gain it back again. What made me think this time would be different?

I felt like a failure. I acted like a failure. I lived like a failure. I set myself up for defeat every time I dieted. I knew what God's Word said, but I had not applied the truth of that Word into my life in such a way that it had transforming power - until now.

The verses from Ephesians rang in my ear. If I were willing to put off my old self and allow Christ to become the center and focus of my life—to renew my mind, to change me from the inside out—then He would develop a plan for my success.

A ray of hope sprang across my soul, and the Lord breathed faith into my weary heart. I did not have to develop a plan. He was doing it for me.

As He stripped off another layer of the old me, I could take the next step. It was time to make an additional adjustment to my mind and attitude. Adjustment is the process of modification.

I looked at the attitudes of the past. I whined and complained about everything. Whatever the subject was, I did not like it, be it the weather or the coffee at the local coffee house. And that was just the beginning. Exercise made me hot and sweaty. I didn't like pain. I even chose a small track near the police station so if I passed out, someone might find me soon enough to get me to the hospital. How I ever gave birth to my children or got to be the size I was I will never understand. I was in some kind of pain all the time—my feet, my knees, my back, my head.

I didn't like any kind of healthy food. Is this a surprise? French fries and ice cream were really my foods of choice. I heard fish was supposed to be good for you, so I stuffed myself with fried catfish. (Was there any other kind?)

And I resented my weight. I was angry at the world, God, and myself. I wanted what I wanted in life, but I wanted it to be easy. Change is not easy—not when we attempt to do it on our own. I believed I did not need to be dependent upon the Lord in order to be successful. No, I could do it on my own. Talk about needing some change. I needed a real attitude of the mind adjustment, and thankfully, the Lord had begun the process.

I asked God for a plan that was attainable and would work for me. So the process began. I gave it a name: the "Step Down" program. I made changes in small steps.

Instead of depriving myself of foods I loved, I modified the way I thought about them. I incorporated thinking about a healthy lifestyle. FP4H calls this "modifying your stinking thinking." The word "diet" always made me feel deprived, so I decided never to use the word again. You can go on and off a diet. A lifestyle is literally a new way of living.

I had to change my old beliefs and stop believing the lies that had held me in bondage and choose to believe the truth. I began the process of taking off the old self (not trying to fix it) and allowing the Lord to change me from the inside out by the renewing of my mind and finally putting on the new self.

My small changes, such as changing to low-fat milk and drinking diet colas knowing I could step down even further later, started adding up to some pretty big results and some very impressive weight loss. I ran the race step by step. I was changing, but I knew I had a long way to go. Would I make the next turn in the race? Some important choices lay ahead. Was I really up to the challenge?

## * Personal Reflection: Change the Mind

Could I make it to the finish line? Yes. But only if I believed the truth that sets me free. I really can "do all things through Christ who strengtheneth me" (Philippians 4:13 KJV). I firmly planted that verse in my mind, but I had to repeat it until it grew in my heart.

Real change began when I allowed the truth of God's Word to make a transformation. Christ is the ultimate source of all truth. When Christ became the center of my life, I found balance and learned to address my problems, including the weight issue, in lasting ways. True and lasting change started in my mind, changing my thought process. The more dependent I became on Christ, the less I depended on myself for the ability to transform my mind.

God's plans work. Lasting change will always start in the mind. We are made new in the attitudes of our minds.

~

# Chapter 3
## Choosing to Change ~ Surrender Willingly

*Sometimes I can hardly see the road in front of me, yet I know I must focus on the path laid out before me. This race is too important to falter now. People line the streets along the course. They wave signs and streamers, ring cowbells, yell, cheer, and encourage me to keep going. "Finish strong!"*

Over the last few years, such words have kept me moving forward.

Sometimes I hear a crowd of supporters scream reinforcement for my change, but I have also heard a small, quiet voice as it whispers across my heart. Just when I think I can't take another step, God sends someone to run alongside me, encourage me, and strengthen me to keep going even when it's hard. "Don't give up," they say. "Focus on the prize. Finish strong. We've got this."

The flip side of encouragement, however, is discouragement. When I see a fellow runner stumble as they try to reach their goal, despair grips my resolve. When I see someone else falter, that frightening word "disaster" brings back memories of failure. *If she fails, will I fail, too?* It's as if in the race we run together, a friend is but a few feet in front of me, when I see her stumble. She is down. Bloody knees and hands push against the hot, uneven asphalt. Tears mixed with sweat stream down her face. I recognize her exhaustion and sense of failure. I've seen it too many times in the mirror. The image of another failed attempt stares at me as memories of every weight-loss program I have tried assault me. *I may fail, too.*

Other racers push past her, their faces showing minimal concern in the heat of the race. As others go on without her, I see the hopeless look on her face. I can see the hopelessness in the slump of her shoulders; I can sense it in the way she hangs her head in defeat. The bystanders scream for her to get up. Wounded and suffering, she surrenders to failure once again. I recognize the surrender because I have experienced that place of defeat. My friend and I had created a cycle of failure in our hearts and minds.

Still the crowd cheers for those left in the race. I hear the voices of friends. "Keep going. Don't stop. Finish strong." Do I keep going or do I stop? What is more important at this point, finishing the race or helping my friend? If I stop to help her and don't finish the race, will I always be someone who loses, who doesn't finish what they start? Surely, if I keep running, someone from the sidelines will come to her aid, but will they understand what these wounds mean to her?

This is a defining moment for me, a crossroad. A choice has to be made. How many times have we encountered such crossroad points when we have to make an important decision? It can be a pivotal circumstance, one that can change the course of our journey. Crossroads are life-changing moments.

I couldn't take my eyes off my fallen friend. I was at a crossroad in the race. How important was finishing? Was the prize really worth it and at what expense? I realized the rest of my journey was dependent on the decision I was about to make. My crossroad stared me in the face and demanded an instant answer. Did I continue or surrender for my friend's sake?

Even though I had only seconds to make my decision, flashes of surrender dashed across my mind, other crossroads of surrender, some forced and some willing. Whether positive or negative surrender, we do not leave the crossroads unchanged.

A couple of old TV shows are great examples of forced surrender and willing surrender.

Back in the late 1950s there was a TV program called *The Roy Rogers Show*. Roy always played the good guy, and of course, there would always be a few bad guys. Roy caught the bad guys and a fight would ensue. The good guys always won. Roy escorted the criminals into jail, usually with their hands raised, and anger embroiled on their faces as they threatened revenge. This is what I call forced surrender. Does this remind you of someone? More than likely, we've all experienced forced surrender.

But not all surrender is forced. I think of another TV show called *The Andy Griffith Show*. If you are familiar with the show, you'll remember Andy Taylor and his son, Opie; the beloved Aunt Bea; and the comical Barney Fife. But do you remember Otis, the town drunk? In a few episodes, Barney put Otis in jail until he could sober up. But in many episodes Otis willingly came into the jailhouse, removed the key from the wall, unlocked the jail cell door, entered the cell, and locked himself in. No one forced Otis into the cell. He came in uncoerced, knowing it was for his own good. Now that is what I would call a willing surrender.

Think about the different aspects of these two types of surrender. The body, attitude, emotions, and mind were all involved in both, but the outcomes were totally different.

So here I was at a crossroad, and I thought of these two types of surrender. I had to make a decision. I had been here before, facing an excuse to falter in my weight-loss journey. I knew how to lose weight, how to get into the race, but the real problem was not starting a race, it was finishing it.

I thought how I had recently broken another barrier and I was almost at the next mile marker. I was less than 280 pounds by now and my plan for change was working. I had a great support group at my church, and I felt better about myself mentally and physically. Losing this weight was the hardest thing I had ever done and finally things really seemed to be working for me. My family was acceptable to the changes I had made, but the truth was I had not really implemented changes for my family. So far, everything had been all about me.

In addition to the stress of losing weight, there were many other pressure points going on in life. My husband and I were in the middle of building a new house, never before having realized the anxiety that would be involved. By the way, if you want to test the strength of your marriage, just build a house together. In addition, we operated a high-pressure and stressful business with long hours on a daily basis. With a change in leadership in our church, we decided to attend a different church. This meant I would no longer be attending the same FP4H class. The new church didn't have a FP4H class, and I thought I couldn't make it without that support group. On top of all of that, I had four teenagers in the house. Do I need to say more?

My brain bounced between the positives and negatives in my life. Life is full of positives and negatives -- good intentions and good excuses. We run along on those good intentions until we encounter a life interruption. What I had to decide was, is this time going to be different? Would I allow the negatives to control the positives? *The crossroad was in front of me, and a decision had to be made.*

Most of us struggle with feelings of inadequacy, yet we insist on fighting battles we cannot win on our own. We fight battles that have already been fought and won when Christ died on the cross. We must learn to surrender our will to the Lord and allow Him to claim battles on our behalf. In the Old Testament, the leader of Israel spoke: "Joshua told the people, 'Consecrate yourselves, for tomorrow the Lord will do amazing things among you'" (Joshua 3:5 NIV). If I followed the command, I needed to consecrate. I needed to commit fully to the Lord and surrender completely and willingly, letting the Lord have control of my life. I had to learn to be an Otis.

To a certain degree, I had surrendered myself to this life-change process, but along with the surrender was a great deal of anger and rebellion. Knowing I needed to lose the weight, my surrender was a forced surrender. I am married to a man who has never had a weight problem. Even though I experienced some success in weight loss, I was angry. It always seemed so unfair.

I tried to see how many French fries I could eat and still be "legal" instead of giving them up entirely because it was the right thing to do. Do you see any resemblance to a forced surrender here?

So I was at the crossroad. I could turn back and once again eat myself into an early grave. I had lost some weight and was feeling better about myself and my health had improved, but my forced surrender had not changed my innermost being. I had been at this same crossroad before. The difference? This time, I could see the crossroad and I knew I needed to surrender—willingly.

Freedom was so close, but then the garbage of lies I had believed stood before me like an overwhelming mountain. The choice had to be made.

Until now, I assumed surrender was a one-time process, but I was wrong. Surrender is a daily process. And some days, surrendering is harder than other days.

If I'm going to be an Otis, I need to participate with the Lord instead of against Him. As my surrender transformed from forced to willing, the first change I noticed was spiritual balance. Spiritual balance isn't the easiest change, but it is the most important.

Negative decisions seemed natural because I had made so many wrong decisions. Spirit-filled decisions seem abnormal to a mind set on defeat and rebellion. God used the hard, dark places and the crossroads to refine me, grow me, make me more like Him. Had I not come through the devastating circumstances of being overweight for the greater part of my life, I wouldn't have experienced deliverance by my Deliverer, healing by my Healer, provision from my Provider, and comfort from my Comforter. It was in the dark place of bondage that I surrendered. God proved His character in these tough places.

In the decisive moments at each crossroad, we can choose to give up and turn around or to remain faithful to the One who helps us through our pain. Quitting often seems easier than finishing. In the early days of my weight-loss journey friends stood by me and wouldn't let me quit. Yes, I had fallen before, but they picked me up, brushed me off, and sent me back out on the track.

For that reason, I am not willing to give up on others now, not even in this race. Because I have changed my surrender from forced to willing, I see different options. Stopping to help others along the way doesn't mean I have to quit. My choice has been made; regardless of my race time, I can still finish.

I choose to stop; help my wounded friend, and put my arm around her waist. If necessary, I will carry her to the finish line. Isn't that what Christ did for me? With a mixture of blood, sweat, and tears staining her precious face I also recognize a spirit of thankfulness and joy. Wholehearted willing surrender to God has at last led me to freedom.

Are you struggling with failure? There is nothing wrong with failing. We all struggle and we all fail at times, but *failure* is another story. Failure happens if we don't get back up. On the road to Golgotha, Jesus stumbled and then fell. What if He hadn't gotten up? Where would you and I be today? He continued His journey. Because of His struggle and His victory at the cross, we are empowered to get up and move forward.

Sometimes we hesitate to continue our journey because we see little or no results. But Christ maintained a heavenly perspective for our future empowerment. We may not see the good that will result from our efforts until later. However, we can claim victory. Paul said, "Be steadfast, immovable, always abounding in the work of the Lord" (1 Corinthians 15:58 NIV). Because of His victory, we can claim victory in all things. When I willingly surrendered, I acknowledged my real success was dependent on a higher power. My victory is dependent upon God.

Anything I hold on to, anything I am unable or unwilling to give over to Him is actually holding on to me. Am I willing to do whatever is necessary to loosen the chains of bondage? What are you holding on to? What is holding on to you? Are you willing to do whatever is necessary to loosen the chains?

Daily I wrestle with desires that take hold of me. Repeatedly, He asks me to give Him full control. Answering Him is tough, but I know I am not going to be truly happy, free, and at peace until I say yes. I am willing to do things His way. I give myself over to willing surrender.

How do you get there? Complete and total surrender; give it over to the loving hands of the Father. Paul said, "Therefore I urge you, brethren, by the mercies of God, to present your bodies a living and holy sacrifice, acceptable to God, which is your spiritual service of worship" (Romans 12:1 NASB).

God requires surrender, as a living sacrifice. Daily we lay aside our own desires to follow Him. Full surrender means we put our energy and resources at His disposal and trust Him to guide us in every detail – even the foods we eat and drink.

Before Jesus gave His life for us, he stopped at Gethsemane. There, He submitted to the will of His Father. Our first stop is our own Gethsemane. To surrender we must say, "Lord, I am giving you full authority in my life."

After submitting His will to God, Jesus freely surrendered to Calvary. Our second stop is our personal Calvary where we give God our surrendered self. Calvary was painful and costly for Jesus, and reaching our goal is also painful and costly, but getting there is priceless. God was after my heart, but He wanted my whole heart not a divided heart. God said, "Man does not see what the Lord sees, for man sees what is visible, but the Lord sees the heart" (1 Samuel 16:17 HCSB).

As I reached to take the arm of my sister along the race, I helped her get up and back on track. I could sense the smile of my heavenly Father. I understood the encouragement, "Keep going, Joyce. Even when it's hard, don't give up. Focus on the prize. Finish strong. Take your sister with you; she is worth the effort and so are you. You are both precious to me."

# * Personal Reflection: Surrender the Attitude

Surrender is a major step for real life change. We cannot continue to be rebellious and angry about change. A positive attitude brings real and lasting life change. We cannot continue to do negative things and expect to get positive results. This is one reason I love the positive affirmations in the back of this book. Use them. They will change your attitude too!

Kathy worked at our church but never participated in FP4H. She thought we sat around and whined about our weight and she did not want to be part of such a thing. One day God whispered into the quiet place of longing in Kathy's heart and began a process of change and surrender. Here is Kathy's story about learning to surrender.

## Kathy Nelson's Surrender

I had always been overweight. In high school I wore a size 14/16. Even at church, among teen friends, I never felt I totally belonged. So many of them were petite, skinny girls, while I was a plump teenager in clothes sizes meant for overweight women. Weight wasn't the only issue. Family economics played into my self-image and I saw myself as the "girl from the wrong side of the tracks." My low self-esteem only fueled my weight problem.

During these teen years, I noticed I was the fat girl and decided to do something about it. I played around with purging; however, I was too scared to do it often. I knew it wasn't the real answer. I believed I wasn't worthy enough for the popular or smart boys I knew, so I dated losers, guys who were going nowhere.

I eventually married one of those losers, excited over the fact that someone wanted me. But our marriage had been wrong from the start. I was looking for something that would boost my self-image and that marriage was not it. Ten and a half months later, the marriage was over. The euphoria of being married and wanted had faded. I failed in my marriage, I failed my parents and disappointed myself. In my mind at that moment; I thought I was destined to be a failure.

I removed myself from all my childhood friends and any activity thing that might hurt me. Then I met Ricky and we were best friends from day one. Ricky and I soon married. My new husband taught me to cook, and his method of cooking was fantastic though we ate a lot of Hamburger Helper, grilled foods covered in every kind of sauce we could find, and Jiffy cornbread. Somehow, I managed to do okay with our food choices.

Then our son Daniel arrived. We were a happy family and I became a stay-at-home mom. Other than chasing a toddler, there wasn't much exercise in my life. The unhealthy eating habits soon caught up with me and my weight increased. I knew I needed to do something.

I met a woman who said she also wanted to lose weight and suggested we join Weight Watchers using a buddy system. I was all in. We started doing well. We ate well all week, then after weigh-in on Thursday nights, we'd stop at Wendy's for a hamburger, fries, and coke. After several more times of getting off program during the week, on Wednesday I ate turnip greens and Raisin Bran (low calorie and high fiber) to clean my system before Thursday night weigh-in. I noticed I wasn't losing weight and turned back to my old trick of purging once again.

The stress of the scales sent me over the edge. This program wasn't working for me, so I quit. I decided to settle with who and how I was. I wasn't happy with myself; I had simply surrendered once again to my old mindset of failure.

The church I attended had some legalistic ideas about the role of women within the church body, which only added to the inadequacies of my self-image. I was a woman. I was a nobody. I had no identity. I was a 235-pound invisible person.

Still, I was Ricky's wife and Daniel's mother. Then in June 1997, Ricky passed away. My whole world was rocked. My only real identity had been as Ricky's wife for so long. Now my grief seemed surreal. I wasn't angry, but I missed my best friend, my husband, and I was broken-hearted for my child. I didn't know what to do with all my emotions. I crammed them inside and refused to let them out. I knew my response wasn't healthy, but I didn't know what else to do. When anyone asked, I said, "I'm great," but I was dying on the inside.

Little by little, my voice grew bolder and my faith matured. I was more than Ricky's wife; I became Kathy. My faith grew because I depended on the Lord to help me. I joined the YMCA and became best friends with the treadmill. I was proud of myself when I was able to speed walk ten miles a week. I didn't know what else to do in the gym, but it was a start.

My eating habits were still not the best and I wasn't adjusting well to cooking for two instead of three. Soon, Daniel and I found regular places to eat out for each night of the week. I didn't stop to think about the poor eating habits I was instilling in my son. All I wanted was to get through each day. I made changes in my body but my mind still hung on to the feelings of not being "good enough." So I pushed myself harder.

In 1999, my weight dropped to 175 pounds. I couldn't believe it. For the first time in my life, I liked who I was becoming. In August of that year, I met Steve, and we hit it off from the start. In May 2000, Steve and I married, which meant a move to another town for Daniel and me.

The move and the marriage were good. God placed us in a wonderful church body. From the moment I walked in the door of the church, I knew something was different. Moving forward, I began to enjoy cooking again, and Steve loved to eat. I remember trying a new recipe once and Steve actually cried. He said it was because it tasted so good, but I don't know if it was that or simply the fact that I was cooking again.

Then it began to happen. I started putting on a little weight. So I resorted to an old trick. Yes, I began purging again. Then I learned that one of my co-worker's daughters had an eating disorder.

Listening to her story, I knew God had brought me to that particular job to save me from a road of destruction with purging. I am aware God had His hand on me, but when I saw Him at work in my life, it became a divine moment.

I stopped purging but continued in my quest to find the perfect diet again. Family members mentioned my weight gain. "Here we go again," I thought, "the 'not good enough syndrome.'" Some family members recommended the Atkins diet, so I tried that. Failed again. I ordered diet pills and I lost some weight; however, it was just for a short season and included some unwelcome side effects. Once again, I went back to Weight Watchers. I was in this horrible cycle of trying not to return to that dreaded 235 pounds, but nothing worked for me. After someone made yet another remark about my weight, I stood in our den screaming at Steve saying, "I can't go through this again."

Then our church started a new session of First Place 4 Health, a Christ-centered weight-loss program. I fought the idea of such a group. I assumed they would be a bunch of women whining about their weight, and I didn't want any part of it. However, I was desperate, and I needed relief from my emotions as well as my weight. Some of my church friends joined the program and I saw them have a certain measure of success. I asked my husband, who is in the medical field, for his opinion of this new diet. He was totally against it but suggested I speak to my doctor.

Finally, I walked into my doctor's office and broke down. I was done. I couldn't take it anymore. I had tried every diet and had overcome an eating disorder. My heart screamed, "Enough already!" I didn't care what form it came in -- a magic pill, diet, or whatever. I needed something to happen that day, yet in reality, I knew my weight problem wasn't going to go away overnight.

As I cried out to my doctor, he listened. Then he encouraged me to make some real lifestyle changes. Finally, I surrendered and signed up for the FP4H Bible study. For the first time in my life, I was doing something for me. This would be a journey about God and me, and weight loss or not, no one would take away my surrender.

I learned early in life that I was created to glorify God. While my mind knew, I had not applied my learning on a personal level. With the Bible study, I began to search for God's purpose for my life. As I transferred from head knowledge to heart attitude, I realized I was created to do great and mighty things. I learned to say, "I am a daughter of the King and I am worthy." I am in a battle on many levels, learning to die to self every day, willingly surrendering to the changes the Lord wants in my life.

In October, I completed my first half marathon. It was one of the most emotional things I have experienced. My friend Brenda and I stayed together for the first twelve miles. With 1.3 miles left, I said, "We need to put music in our ears and push. Let's run hard and give it all we have." So the last mile, it was just God, worship music, and me. Charles Billingsley sang "Marks of a Mission" and "Finish Strong."

I topped the hill crossing Main Street. A policeman stopped traffic and waved me across the four-lane intersection. At that moment, the world stopped to let me pass and I cried. So often in life, I had wondered if Jesus would notice me in a crowd of people. Today, it seemed He said to me, "I see you, Kathy, and I've stopped the world just for you."

Recently, I found an old picture of myself and I cried. The picture was taken about the time my husband Ricky passed away, but the woman in the photograph no longer looked like me. I have changed physically and on so many other levels. The more I am willing to surrender, the more God changes my life.

So far, I have lost fifty-five pounds. I'll reach my goal weight when I lose twelve more pounds. I have invited God along on my journey. He has transformed every area of my life -- physical, emotional, mental, and most importantly, spiritual. My life belongs to Him. He has so much for me. I am reminded of the song "This Little Light of Mine." The children's song is now my theme song.

In everything I do, I surrender to His will. Jesus knew the will of the Father, and Jesus could have called down a legion of angels to save Him, but He surrendered willingly. God has had His hand on me every step of the way. Nothing touches my life until it passes through His hands.

Surrender has not been an easy or a pretty thing, but I have now found peace and joy in surrendering my will to His. One day I shall stand before my King and hear Him say, "Well done, my daughter." At the end of my journey, I want to be able to say, "With Your help, I did it."

Note from Joyce: As we go to publication, Kathy has accomplished her goal weight. God is truly awesome.

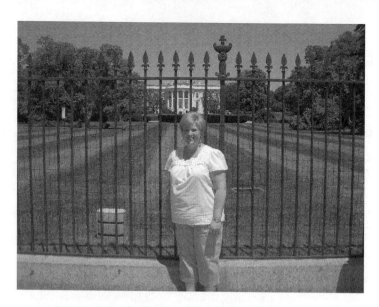

Kathy Nelson Before Picture--May of 2010

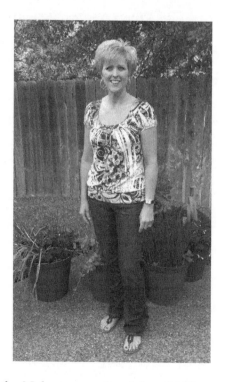

Kathy Nelson at goal weight of 138 pounds

~

# Chapter 4

## Preparing for the Race ~ Train the Body and Soul

*I just stepped past another runner and I can tell this race is harder on some than others. It is evident in the slower pace I see in other participants as I move ahead one step at a time. There is another bend in the road up ahead. I catch a glimpse of the finish line, but it is as if I am never going to make it. I am so tired. I knew this leg of the race today would be difficult. I had prepared for this time and place. Every runner does. (By the way, my friends would not call me a real runner. I am more a walker/runner.) Regardless, training and practice are necessary for success in running a marathon, in developing a fitness program and even for a weight-loss plan. I learned this the hard way.*

I have seen all kinds of runners. Some sign up for a race, buy a new pair of running shoes, and start training. They work out the details of the training plan. They start strong. Then one day they have to work late or days get busy and then they miss a training session or two. They tell themselves that at least they are making some effort to train. On race day they show up, start solid. Halfway through the race, they develop a leg cramp or run out of energy. Some runners call it being gassed. They quit, frustrated and disappointed with themselves.

Other runners start training, run a few times, and quit. They never make it to the race. In both cases, something distracted them from the plan (if there was a plan at all). This start-stop-quit is the way I approached weight loss in the past. Without proper planning and training, we are unable to build the endurance we need to run and finish.

With accurate training, we can prepare for and overcome obstacles in every leg of a weight-loss race whether the obstacle is mental, emotional, or physical.

Planning and preparation are not foreign to most people. Don't most of us have life insurance of some kind? Politicians plan and prepare for years with the single thought of being voted into an office. When our children are born, we begin preparing for them to attend high school, college, and then leave the nest. We even plan our vacations. We map out the route, how long it should take, where we will be staying, and what we will do when we arrive.

My weight-loss journey was no different. In the early days, I don't think I realized the importance preparation played in attaining achievement. Preparing is a vital key to success and to finishing. My FP4H leader said, "If you fail to plan, you are planning to fail." Preparation comes in levels; as my body became adjusted to the new eating plan and the new routine and amount of exercise, then the level, intensity, or type of exercise was modified to train further, to endure more, and be stronger. I re-adjust my training plan about every ten to fifteen pounds of weight loss.

Preparing and planning are kind of like peanut butter and jelly; they go hand in hand, as do food and exercise. One supports the other. Doing one without the other may allow us to see some short-term results, but if long-term, life-changing results are the goal, we need proper and balanced combinations.

Some people are natural-born planners and list makers. If you are a planner, bless your heart (as we say in the South). And then there are the rest of us. I am, by nature, a spontaneous person, operating off the hip, as my husband would say. I have learned to plan and be a list maker, not easy for a free-hearted, fun-loving girl, but with the Lord's help I now plan and prepare.

As I studied the book of Nehemiah during my daily Bible reading time, a couple of key points made a real impact on me. Nehemiah planned his rebuilding of the wall in Jerusalem by assessing the damage and developing a realistic strategy. He kept the plan simple and took quick action. He was not swayed by what others thought. He planned his work and worked his plan. Nehemiah constantly combined prayer with preparation. Success requires the risk of failure, and rewards involve hard work. Nehemiah's plan and system sounds like a FP4H session!

I also learned from Nehemiah that a plan and hard work will encounter opposition. But when problems arose, he prayed for the Lord to strengthen his hands. This revelation had a major impact on me. I had hoped my journey to lose weight would be easy. I was a busy woman, working, taking care of my kids, and serving at my church. Honestly, it was easier to let things happen. When I had a bad week, I could blame it on circumstances of life.

Nehemiah didn't look for excuses. When things got tough for Nehemiah, he asked the Lord to strengthen him. He showed me a glimpse of tremendous determination and character to remain steadfast. I was still looking for someone else to blame. I realized the Lord had prepared me for the journey. It was time for me to take a risk and leave the excuses behind.

Paul said, "Remember this: Whoever sows sparingly will also reap sparingly, and whoever sows generously will also reap generously" (2 Corinthians 9:6 NIV). And the writer of Hebrews said, "...he [God] rewards those who earnestly seek him" (Hebrews 11:6 NIV).

A solid plan will yield abundant rewards in all aspects of my life, provided I am willing to do my part. Likewise, I could not expect to reap long-lasting benefits of continued weight loss if I was not willing to do hard work and some serious planning. It was time for me to sow generously. It was time for me to invest time and effort into this new lifestyle.

Deep in my heart and soul, I longed for freedom from the extra weight. Though I had cried out to the Lord to free me many times, now I took a good, hard look in the mirror. Two hundred fifty pounds called my name and I felt I could not settle for less than the next mile marker. I had to make the next mile in the race. No more excuses. The Lord captured my heart, and I did not want to accept changes in weight loss alone. I wanted life change.

I started with a yearly plan, but now I do a new planning session every three months. Remember, people who do not plan, plan to fail. My first step was to look at the food I ate. I am a picky eater. My friends often made fun of me because I owned a produce company yet did not like any kind of vegetables, especially anything green. So instead of whining about what I did not like, I adopted the principles of the sound eating plan of FP4H. I started adding foods I liked to eat and foods I needed to try.

These additions sounded simple but were not. I did it because it was the right thing to do, not because I wanted to. I believed eating right would eventually become my new normal. I could not wait for my "wants" to change. I modified types and amounts of foods I ate. I called my new plan my "step-down" program. I will explain it fully in a later chapter.

As I worked on my food plan, I made specific decisions. Rather than saying I would eat better, I wrote down what I would and would not eat. I gave up fried foods because it was an area of slavery and I needed to be free of it. I was addicted to French fries and I knew it. (About once a month, I allowed myself to eat something fried. I continue this reward concept in my overall plan). I planned my family's meals and grocery lists around having at least five fresh vegetables and fruits a day.

As I continued tweaking my plan, I asked questions. Is this meal balanced? Am I eating as healthy as possible? Am I eating from all the food groups? Am I eating a proper portion? Small changes, those baby steps, made a big difference for me.

My weight dropped to about 240 pounds, which was better than I expected. My little changes were having a big impact. My doctor was proud; at this point he took me off blood pressure medicine, and then encouraged me to keep losing.

I lost enough weight that others were beginning to notice. I loved it when someone noticed and felt proud of my weight loss, but I needed more than a food plan; I needed exercise. I remember the first time I went to a local walking track. Walking was not one of my favorite activities; in fact, I hated it. I forced myself to walk one lap around the track—a quarter of a mile. It was difficult, and I thought I would have a heart attack. I didn't. The best I could do that first night was one lap. The next evening I did it again, and then day after day, again and again. Soon I could walk four laps—a whole mile.

I kept going until I was up to two miles, then three. You'd think by now I would be elated and had learned to enjoy walking, but I still hated it. Like it or not, I kept going back to that little track. I was determined to follow my plan to include some type of exercise every day, six days a week.

A day came when I failed to make it to the track. In the past I would have beat myself up or given up, but not this time. I started walking around my coffee table. Around and around and around. If that sounds crazy, don't worry, my family thought so, too.

My family didn't embrace the weight loss or the exercise, and discussing anything about weight had become taboo. My husband tried to be supportive. He participated grudgingly in this new lifestyle, but he had no plans to join me in exercising. Maybe it was because he had seen me go through the weight loss and gain cycle many times before.

He said the right things. He loved me as I had been before and loved me as I was now. And while I needed his love and support, I also needed a team partner rather than an enabler. He had never had a weight problem in his life. I don't think he knew exactly what to do. I needed my journey to become a team journey, something for our entire family, not just for me.

Following a daily and weekly plan for food preparation and exercise took up a great deal of valuable time. It took away time from family, work, and church activities. As I incorporated time for my new lifestyle, I felt guilty. I never wanted to go back to food for comfort, so I had to look elsewhere for how I could deal with my guilt.

The Lord took me back to the book of Nehemiah. In chapters six and seven, Nehemiah did not have the full support of the people he served. People told him the rebuilding of the wall could not be accomplished; it was too great a task and could not be done. Nehemiah could have succumbed to guilt, feeling that he was wasting his time. But he didn't.

A warning bell went off in my head. The powerful Word of the Lord helped me understand there was no room for guilt when following His plan. My job was to focus on the work at hand and follow through with the task He had given me.

The next afternoon I enlisted my husband's help. I placed my hands on each side of his face and in my sweetest voice possible, I said he needed to get on my team or get out of my way. I told him how much I loved him but I needed him to be my biggest fan. If he couldn't, I had to keep going. I had to finish. That day was a turning point. My husband joined my team and with his support, I began to see other positive changes in my family as well.

During the time of Nehemiah, Israel was devastated by times of intense rebellion and sin, yet when the people repented and returned to God, He delivered them. As I read Israel's story, I realized my weight issue had a name – rebellion and sin. How many times had I walked the weight-loss road looking for mercy? God had been there all the time and willing to help, but until now, I had never been willing or ready to make the changes in my attitude and behavior that would correct the situation.

The book of Nehemiah was about rebuilding the wall of a great city, but it was also about the spiritual renewal and rebuilding of a people's dependence on God. More important, the book of Nehemiah was about me. Rebellion and sin versus attitude and behavior.

God peeled back the next layer in the life-change process. There would be a couple of detours before I could claim the finish line as mine. What I did not realize was how close they really were. They were just up ahead. Was I really ready? We all take detours, but it's how we come out on the other side that counts. My detours made me wonder.


## * Personal Reflection: Plan for Success

When we fail to plan, then we plan to fail. There never has been a truer statement made. I know I could not have been successful without a plan. We are all human and imperfect individuals. I needed training and practice to achieve a solid plan. To accomplish this I had to develop a thoughtful and practical step-by-step plan for weight-loss success.

Not only did planning help me become more efficient with my busy schedule, it also kept me committed to following through on my long-term goals. Getting the weight off was the first challenge; keeping the weight off is the ultimate challenge. The plan had to include a food and exercise program because success would not be long-term without both components - kind of like peanut butter and jelly.

When Donna first joined one of our classes, I commented that I love exercise. Donna raised her hand and said, "I don't get that. I hate exercise." I told her to stick around for the next twelve weeks and she would "get it." She did finally understand. But that is not all she got. Here is Donna's story.


## Donna Conerly ~ Running by Faith

The beginning of "Real Life Change" for me began in January 2009. A friend and I decided to attend a FP4H Bible study. Both of us had tried multiple weight-loss tactics and we figured, what did we have to lose? (ha-ha). I weighed 189 pounds and stood five foot three.

As a nurse, I was not really motivated in the first few weeks of the program. I told my friend, "We already know this stuff; we just need to do it." I faithfully completed my Bible study and attended the class each week. In class, I listened and learned the program and did my best to follow the guidelines as they were taught to me. I also started to exercise five days a week (which I hated at the time). I walked fifteen to twenty minutes a day, gradually increasing my time and distance as I became more cardio fit. In the thirteen weeks of session one, I lost 19.2 pounds. I immediately signed up for session two. In between sessions, I attended an accountability class. I didn't want to break the pace I set for myself.

You see, I was scared. I knew me. I had lost weight so many times before and gained it back, with a little extra to go with it. Accountability kept me in sync. I lost 3.4 pounds in between sessions. Then in session two, I worked even harder. I completed my Bible study each day and began to pray more. I asked God to help me stay on track. I listened. I learned more about the program and understood some of the principles taught in the food sessions. I asked questions and participated in class; I shared some of my fears and difficulties and some of my successes. I continued to exercise by walking and even incorporated some "trotting" into my walks. In session two, I lost 14.2 pounds in thirteen weeks. Within twelve months, I lost 45.2 more pounds and reached my goal weight of 130 pounds. Praise the Lord. I owe all honor and glory to Him.

The Lord and I together have managed to keep the weight off for twenty-one months and counting. The pounds lost are great. Am I happy? Yes. But the most fantastic transformation took place in my heart and my mind. The Holy Spirit pierced my heart, setting me free from the bondage of food and the powerful hold and ungodly place I had given it in my life. You see, my blinders were removed and I finally admitted I was living in sin and food was my idol. Christ was not first in my life, food was.

I am free from the burden, which I had lived under most of my adult life. Today, at age fifty-two, Christ is first in my life. I wake daily to bring honor and glory to Him in all I do and say, including what I choose to eat. Yes, He cares what I eat. He cares how I nourish, exercise, and care for this physical body--the temple in which His Spirit lives.

He also gave me the desire to make a life change rather than continue to live on a diet plan. There are some of you who think, "Good grief, just tell me how you lost the weight." Here are a few reasons I am successful. First, I admitted my addiction to food and asked God to help me break free from my sin of overeating and lack of concern in caring for my body, His temple.

Next, I was consistent. I learned the program, practiced the principles of FP4H, never missed class, and never quit—even in between sessions. Am I going to do this program for the rest of my life? You bet. I sure am. It's a real life change for me. I'm in forever. I never want to go back to being overweight. I have learned to be mindful and intentional and to make right choices every day. I have also learned to forgive myself when I make poor choices, and I continually strive to do the next right thing.

The Lord has done several other great things in my life over the last two years, including bringing me a wonderful husband. After being single for more than sixteen years, Mike and I met, and he joined the FP4H program with me. We also married. That's right, and you know what else is great about that? We have become best friends. We work out together and train together, and Mike loves to cook. So making healthy choices at our house is natural.

Mike and I have run several marathons together. The Lord also has given us great friends to hang out with that have become our training partners, accountability partners, and mentors. I am so thankful God brought me to First Place 4 Health. I'm forever changed and strengthened by the program. I am thankful also for the close bond of friendship and accountability the program has given me. I draw strength and encouragement from my FP4H friends.

I will end my story with something I am now very passionate about: exercise. Remember earlier, I told you I hated it? Well, God changed that, too. I have always been very competitive and I love a challenge. In session two, I incorporated "trotting" into my walking routine. Well, my trotting slowly turned into jogging, and now I am able to actually run. To date, I have finished two full marathons (26.2 miles), five half-marathons (13.1 miles), two 12Ks (7.46 miles), and several 5Ks (3.1 miles). I love running, and joy fills my body and soul as I run and even more when I race.

As the starting gun fires, my feet begin to move at the pace I have trained for. I enjoy running. I enjoy my heart pumping at a rate that makes it grow stronger and stronger. I love the rapid rush of blood through my body as all my vessels expand from the pressure and heat created as I run. I love the shortness of breath as my lungs work to force necessary oxygen to mix with my blood so I can survive the run, the tightness of my muscles conserving energy needed for the endurance to finish strong. But most of all I love the clarity of my mind as I run. Every race is different, just as in life. We each have our own journey. The key is to listen and obey.

I love training and preparing for races. It helps me stay focused. I love to set goals for myself and strive to attain them one by one. Running and preparing for races is a lot like life. I must prepare to run my best race. I must take in good quality foods to fuel my physical body. I must have good shoes and use my Garmin and heart-rate monitor to help me meet my goals. In life, I must feed on God's Word daily to gain strength, knowledge, and wisdom to withstand the enemy and all the fiery darts he will fire at me. I must armor up every day.

I train consistently to stay fit, and I add strength training into my workouts. In life, I attend church regularly (iron sharpens iron). I become stronger when my husband and running buddy, family, and close friends encourage me and hold me accountable. Attending Bible studies, taking mission trips, and serving in my church and community strengthen me.

Rest is also super important. For my physical body to run and perform at its best I must get the proper amount of physical rest. In life, we need time to rest, reflect, and revive our spirits. We need to spend time alone with our Heavenly Father and draw close to Him.

Enjoy the race. Know your pace. Run your race. In life, enjoy your journey. God has a specific purpose and plan just for you. Don't worry about Sally Sue. Pray for her to run her race and enjoy her journey, but you focus on what God intends for you. My prayer for you as you continue this book is that you will be encouraged and inspired to get up and get in the race and that you will run your best race possible, consistently staying on pace.

All 4 Him,
Donna Conerly

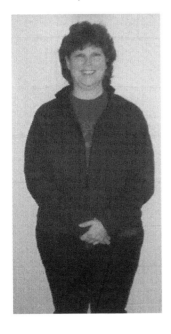

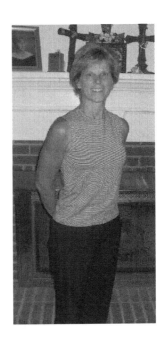

Donna Conerly January 2009          Donna Conerly at goal weight

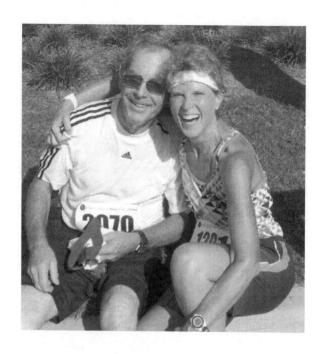

Mike and Donna Conerly after half-marathon (one of many)

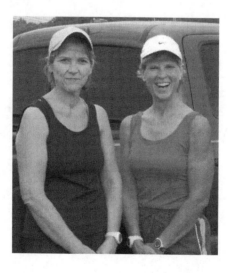

Donna and Joyce in training for half-marathon

~

## Chapter 5
## Detours ~ Journey Through the Desert

*Race officials announced a change in the course. During the previous night, a water main beneath the street had burst due to age and increased pressure. (I kind of sympathized with that old water line and jokingly told my friends that sounded like many of us. How many times under pressure do we fold, give in, and give up?) The announcer explained that even though repair crews had worked through the night, the broken water main was still un-repaired. Our route had been altered and racers would be directed via a detour around the problem.*

*At mile twelve, the detour signs appeared. Detour ahead. My training partner stepped beside me and quietly reminded me not to be anxious or lose pace. She had pushed me at times over the last few months, past my normal endurance level, past what I thought I could bear. She had helped train me for unexpected issues like we were encountering today. Training for months was about to pay off at this unexpected detour as we pushed toward the finish line.*

Life often comes with detours. Some detours come with warnings to alert me of pending danger. Others seem to appear by surprise with no advance warning. Sometimes I have chosen to make my own way due to my stubbornness or rebellion. Sometimes God allows distractions and diversion to grow me into more than I could ever imagine. Regardless of the type of detour, we have all experienced them.

Detours can be short and minor while others are long, deep, and painful, and cause us to doubt others and ourselves.

Sometimes a detour is so devastating we wonder how much more we can take and cry out in anguish for help. Some detours are like rivers that are fast flowing and almost take us under the raging current. Others are deserts that cause us to wander around in circles and in the process, we realize how dry and parched we are. Detours throw us off course and many times they throw us off pace. They can cause us to miss the finish line.

Challenges, changes, and choices lace our journey each day. And, yes, there will be detours. The dictionary says a detour is a deviation from a direct course of action. A detour can be for the benefit of a person's conduct, job, or calling in life. A detour can be for our betterment and improvement.

There was a time when I took detours simply because I chose to go my own way and didn't really care how it would affect others or me in the future. Pure rebellion is a simple term I don't really like, but it applies to many of the detours in my life. The way we each navigate our journey and the detours we take have lasting consequences on our life and on the lives of others. Like it or not, our choices matter.

Sometimes detours make us lose pace and falter in our rate of speed. We may still be moving but at an altered pace. Sometimes I must purposely alter my pace to continue to the finish line. This is a sign of growth and maturity. Training partners and co-workers remind me to pace myself. And thankfully, the Lord, too, prompts me to pace myself as He guides me through tough spots.

Many times, I have set goals for myself that push me past my limits. In races, I have lost my pace, faltered, and sustained injuries. The extent of an incorrect pace determines how quickly I recover when I hit a detour. God wants me to reach my full potential, but He doesn't ask me to go beyond the pace He sets for me.

Detours not only alter our physical pace but also change emotional and spiritual pace. Being aware of detours helps me navigate the future because detours will come as we continue our race for the Lord.

Detours that come with warning signs are not as difficult for me as the ones that take me by surprise. Unexpected detours cause a more drastic change in pace. After losing 113 pounds, I was pumped. I could see the 200-pound mark as a doable goal. I was eating right, exercising, and progressing at a good pace. I started leading a FP4H class at my church and felt on track in all areas. Leading the group gave me the accountability I needed and the spiritual growth that was important for a well-balanced plan. Then I hit several unpredicted detours.

The first surprise detour came when a special friend suddenly moved away. The Lord had brought us together and we became the closest of friends and partners in teaching class. We worked out together, studied together, challenged each other to make our personal goals, rooted each other on in good times, and helped each other in the down times. She challenged me to sign up for my first half marathon. We rejoiced as we crossed the finish line in that race. We became true sisters in the life-change process. And then she moved away.

I was not prepared for the loss. I had depended on her so much and when she was gone, I struggled to find my pace again. I was lonely and so emotionally disappointed that I wanted to give up, quit, and not finish. My emotional pain sidetracked me from my original goals. Have you ever experienced this kind of aimlessness? Maybe for you it was the loss of a spouse to death or divorce. Maybe it was the loss of a parent, a job, a child, or a special friend. Maybe it was a devastating injury or illness. The common denominator for all detours is pain, and pain throws us off pace.

A second surprise detour rocked my world when a tornado ripped through Magee, Mississippi. My precious parents, both in their seventies, had already weathered Hurricane Katrina a few years prior. Now an EF3 tornado struck the north part of their city. The tornado significantly damaged the town's water treatment plant, interrupting service to the entire town. The tornado also destroyed sixty homes. One of those homes belonged to my parents.

They lost much that day but were blessed to be alive. The physical destruction was overwhelming, but the emotional devastation was the real detour for me. I sat in Mom and Dad's front yard and ate a gallon-size bag of homemade chocolate chip cookies. One cookie was not enough. I cried, ate a cookie, cried, ate a cookie, cried some more, until I was totally emotionally spent.

The cookies were soon gone, but the destruction was still there. My fix for the detour had not met the needs of the day. After the storm of tears and cookies, I felt worse than ever. I had heard of people falling off the wagon, but I was not only off the wagon, I was knee-deep in mud. But God knew where I was, and after the emotional detour of wind, cookies, and tears, He reached down and loved me, mud and all. He not only loved me, but through many Christians, family, friends, and some strangers, He loved the town of Magee, including my parents and our entire family.

Keep in mind, some detours we take are not for our benefit but for the benefit of others. My cookie detour right after the tornado was a tough place for me personally, but God used that terrible tornado as a catalyst in my family.

A few years before the tornado, my folks began attending a small church near their home. Dad knew about Jesus, but he did not know Jesus. Dad had never attended church much, even though Mama was a regular. Dad's work was his excuse, and he felt Jesus surely understood. Mama was so happy. My husband, Glenn, and I prayed for Dad and took every opportunity to share with him the difference in knowing about (head knowledge) and knowing (heart knowledge).

After the tornado destroyed their home, possessions, and almost their lives, the church people showed up with concern, prayers, and practical help for the cleanup and rebuilding. The kindness and love from those people touched my dad's heart. Jesus reached through the hard surface of my dad's heart. At age seventy-six, Dad accepted Jesus into his heart. He came face to face with the Savior in the actions of others, and Dad's life was changed forever.

The devastation I saw as a detour God used as an everlasting change for Dad. On a Sunday night not too long ago in a small church in Magee, Mississippi, along with my four sisters and only brother, I watched Dad be baptized. Dad said, "I have needed a bath a long time, but I am clean now." Yes, Daddy, you are. White as snow all because God our Father decided to send His beloved Son to this earth as a baby so that one day He could go to a cross so that we might have eternal life. The love of our Heavenly Father amazes me. It is never too late, nor are we too old to experience the life-changing touch of the Savior.

Was the tornado detour worth it? Absolutely. I didn't see it the day I cried and ate the bag of cookies, but I can see it now in the eyes of my daddy. What a sweet reflection I see.

Shortly after the speed bump detour of the Magee tornado, my husband's brother Jimmy lost his battle with lung cancer. My husband was a year older than Jimmy, and he never expected to lose his younger brother. Life wasn't supposed to happen that way.

In the midst of our grief, I watched the daily downward spiral of Glenn's mother. Frances had lived with us for four and a half years. She suffers from Alzheimer's. We all love her and try to show her how much we care, but her mind does not remember and her eyes are vacant. She has no recognition of the ones she loves the most. Even though I see patches of recognition and understanding, watching her health deteriorate was and is a painful detour.

We take so much in life for granted, and when a detour occurs, we struggle with all the emotions we experience in the process. We cry out to God, "Why? Why me? Why now? Why this?" Detour signs and surprise detours will always be just ahead. It is what we do during and after the detours that will mark the difference in the life-change process.

Our journey, including the detours, the twists and turns, the hills and valleys, and even people and places impact and define our life stories. So often, we focus on making big changes that we think can make a difference quickly.

Unfortunately, at times these changes are not lasting. Yet we ignore small daily changes we can make, which over time add up to big transformations that are permanent.

The Israelites are an example of how we sometimes try to handle our detours. During the time of Moses, the Israelites lived under Egyptian rule in bondage as slaves for more than 400 years. God directed Moses to return to Egypt and free His people. The goal was to lead the Israelites out of slavery and into the Promised Land. But Moses and his team didn't get far when they realized Pharaoh and his armies were right behind them. The Israelites were trapped, mountains and hills on both sides, Pharaoh's army gaining on them, and the Red Sea directly in front of them. The plan for freedom wasn't looking too good. The Israelites didn't just lose pace; they were stalled with no visible way out of their predicament.

My cookie binge trapped me, too. Not just off the wagon but in the mud, not sure how to get up. I had to have help beyond my own ability to get back on track and pace.

The Israelites were not prepared for the detour ahead. Their focus had been on freedom from slavery. Now as a roadblock obstructed the path, they cried out thinking they had been better off as slaves. Even though the Israelites experienced great victory when God's powerful hand delivered them from Egypt, their only response now in this hard place was fear, complaining, and despair. I can relate. I sounded just like them, and you may sound like them as well. Just as the Israelites displayed a lack of faith in God's ability, I did the same thing.

God taught me some vital lessons about trust and dependence, which became a catalyst in my life-change process. God also brought me to my knees in desperation and directed me to new strength and understanding. As He guided me through the story of Moses and the Israelites in Exodus 14, the Lord helped me through some tough detours that year.

Those detours are now a continual beacon for me because I need His power to deal with the detours and life interruptions that stop me in my tracks, throw me off pace, and cause me to falter.

In Exodus 14, God prepared Moses, a frail person with flaws, and transformed him into a man of strength. With God's guidance Moses performed great and mighty works. Moses was an outstanding personality shaped by God. Moses had a positive attitude and he called upon the Lord for direction and strength. Moses prayed diligently, sought out God's plan, and when God said move, Moses moved, even when he could not see the path ahead.

The day the Israelites were boxed in with nowhere to turn, God performed one of the greatest miracles of history. With no apparent way of escape, the Lord swept the sea back by a strong east wind and the Israelites crossed over on dry ground. The path was revealed to them and for them at God's perfect timing. Pharaoh's army, breathing down their necks, followed, but was destroyed by the same divine power. God demonstrated His great provision and love for His people that day. Moses learned to react correctly to detours. Holding pace is difficult and so is getting back on track, but it is possible.

My year of detours revealed how I needed to develop a pattern of consistent obedience to God when I was in the easy places, the high roads, and not under great stress and pressure. When I hit the detours and the stress mounts, my natural reaction will be to trust and obey God even when I cannot see the path ahead. I learned to train for detours so that as they come I can adjust my pace, remain consistent, do the right things, and trust God to continue to run the race beside me. Like my training partner who ran beside me in the marathon, He never runs ahead of me or behind me but right next to me. He is pacing me, just as a pacer paces the runners in a marathon.

We all experience detours, but how long we stay sidetracked will depend on how much preparation we have given our plan. Detours are a natural part of life, but our reaction and the decisions and changes we make depend on the type of detour and how we handle it. Some of the changes are hard, painful, and sad, while others are wonderful. Detours will cause us to wonder, doubt, struggle, and re-evaluate what is important in our lives.

I prepared for the race, but the broken water main altered the path. I saw the sign flashing in front of me: "Detour Ahead." God reminded me that I had trained for such detours. I moved around the detour sign; I held my pace. My best friend (yes, God sent me another one), ran beside me, and we paced each other.

God's Word and the principles within will help you keep running the race, detour and all. His principles are worth living by.

Now step forward and let's get moving. We have a race to win. The next mile marker is just ahead. I can just about see my Promised Land.

## * Personal Reflection: Face the Detours

Detours are inevitable. Learning to pace ourselves and recovering quickly is critical for the continuation of the journey. Train so you are prepared for detours. Even if you falter, you can get back on pace and move forward. Do the things you know to do and have trained to do. Focus on the prize ahead, not on the detour. Don't quit. Get back up. Stopping is not an option. Stumbling happens, but we always get to choose to get back up.

Two of my FP4H friends, Keeli O'Cain and Teresa Russell, faced detours. I hope their stories will help, encourage, and inspire you when you face a detour.

# Keeli O'Cain ~ Up the Hill and Around the Bend

When I heard about a weight-loss class my church was offering, I knew it would be my "get skinny" quick fix. During my first session of FP4H, I realized the program was going to be about more than losing weight; it would be a lifestyle change. If I am to lose weight and keep it off, I must give Christ first place in all areas of my life. Sounds simple, doesn't it? However, surrender and obedience were not words I liked to use, especially in reference to myself.

I am a perfectionist and like to be in control of most situations. Along with my perfectionism, I am also obsessive and compulsive. Due to my childhood upbringing and my early adult years, I have struggled with feelings of inadequacy and failure. I want to be in control and perfect. There is only one perfect person and His name is Jesus. FP4H was about to help me encounter Him in a real and lasting way.

I lost some weight and felt great about it, but I also learned there is a difference in knowing about Jesus and knowing Jesus in my heart. Jesus wanted me to surrender and be obedient not because I was supposed to but because I loved Him so much.

My perfectionism struggles caused countless issues in my life. I used food to comfort me through trials and problems. Through First Place, I discovered I am not called to be skinny or perfect. His goal for me is far greater than weight loss. God said, "Call to me and I will answer and reveal to you wondrous secrets that you haven't known" (Jeremiah 33:3 NIV).

The answer to every question and every situation is Jesus. He answers and provides. When I tried to be in control of my situations, I made a bigger mess. Through the power of the words in the Jeremiah verse and help from my First Place group, I began to surrender my will and give up control.

God blessed me in awesome ways. I lost fifty-one pounds and 22 ¾ inches. I began helping with leadership in my FP4H class. I developed strong friendships, studied God's Word. I began to make real and lasting changes in my personal life - from the inside out.

Though not at the finish line, I was running in the right direction. When my FP4H leader asked me to consider serving as a group leader, I was surprised. "Me?"

She said, "God does not call the equipped but equips the called." I was afraid but happy to serve. The old fears rose up and I worried about failing.

Some family issues frustrated me. Then it happened: Detour ahead! I should have seen the warning signs. I was reared in a home where material things and money were at the top of the priority list. As a child, I felt inadequate and never measured up to the standard expected by my mother. Each time I failed, fear of failure grew bigger. I never seem to get anything right, and my mother would show up and fix whatever was wrong. She took control. Her money became a tool to rescue me when I failed. Now I know she was trying to help, but then I felt Mother controlled my life with her money. She meant to help, but each time she corrected my mistakes, my heart suffered wounds and my mind told me I would never measure up to the standard my parents expected.

As a troubled and confused teen, and then as a sad and disheartened young mother trying her best to make a bad marriage survive, I failed again. A broken marriage and wounded children all contributed to my fear of never measuring up.

Then as an adult now in my forties I married my present husband, Donald. I worked in the family business and tried to raise a blended family of five children—mine, his, and ours. Blended families struggle. We sure did. Donald was not a believer and being unequally yoked prevents couples from seeing eye-to-eye on family matters such as raising children and discipline.

It seemed every time there was even a minor disagreement, my mother showed up at the door to take control.

In the middle of all this chaos, I desperately wanted to serve God totally and completely. FP4H had begun to help me build a new foundation, but fear, failure, and frustration at home worked against me.

No wonder I defaulted back to the comfort of food. Personal and family issues sent me on a detour. I was spiritually sidetracked and lost my focus. I stepped back into the bondage of food and reverted to the old lifestyle. I stepped away from all things Jesus, including FP4H. I stopped going to church, having quiet time, praying, and food became my friend again.

Within about five months, I gained twenty-six pounds. I searched my closet for bigger sizes, but I had given all those big clothes away. Reality set in. I was missing more than a few big-sized clothes. I heard the still, quiet voice of the Lord, "You can keep eating and eating, but food will never fill the place that belongs to me in your heart."

He reached out to me even though my sin of disobedience had broken our close relationship. He offered the way back on a road paved with His unconditional love. I had surrendered, but through the tough detour, God showed me a new level of surrender.

Detours aren't easy. My detour tore away at the very foundation of who I thought I was. My journey is filled with uphill climbs and low valleys. Neither uphill climbs nor low valleys are out of His reach. God used my detour to make major repair work in my family and home.

I made the first step back to the path of restoration and healing by trusting God with everything. My husband, my children, my family struggles, my job, my finances, and my future. I could not see the road ahead or where it was leading, but I totally trusted the One who now held my hand.

That pathway included steps back into my quiet time every morning. I spend daily time with God, praying without ceasing, and I've returned to church and FP4H. Both my church and FP4H welcomed me back with open arms of love, not condemnation or judgment.

I am so thankful God uses detours for His glory and purpose. I needed to find my identity in Him before I could move on to His goal for me.

My husband, Donald, has now accepted Jesus as his Lord and Savior, and our children are beginning to experience real and lasting balance in our family. I no longer work in my family's business. I love being a stay-at-home mom. I am learning to trust and allow my husband to lead and guide our family financially. God is also healing and restoring many areas of my life including my children and parents. The work is not complete, but we are moving in the right direction.

I am now back on track to my weight-loss goal - eighteen pounds from my goal weight of 144 pounds. I keep a picture of my beginning weight of 207 pounds as a steady reminder of how far God has brought me. It is also a great reminder every time I want to default back to my old habits and hang-ups. Sixty-three pounds makes a big difference, but the mental and emotional baggage I have dropped weighed so much more and cannot be measured on a set of scales.

Tracking my food and daily exercise are critical for my continued success in this journey. I set new and challenging goals as I continue toward goal weight. I completed my third 5K (and beat my own personal time) and will do a race each month this year. My long-range goal is to make goal weight in the next few months, complete a half-marathon, continue to grow in my spiritual walk as I serve and lead in the FP4H ministry, and most of all I want to allow Jesus to be the center and focus of my life and my family.

I now choose to spend time with Jesus. I surrender to His call on my life daily, sometimes hourly. I will not live on a diet for the rest of my life. I am free to eat any food I want; however, I make better choices because I know my body is the temple of the Holy Spirit. I want to give God my best every minute. Do I sometimes make poor choices? Yes, I do, but I ask God to forgive me and help me with future choices. Then I get right back on track!

My weight loss is only an outward sign of the greater internal work God has done.

Keeli O'Cain, Pelahatchie, Mississippi

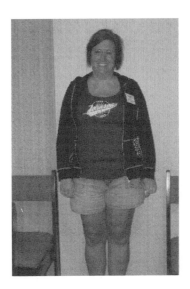

Keeli O'Cain Before

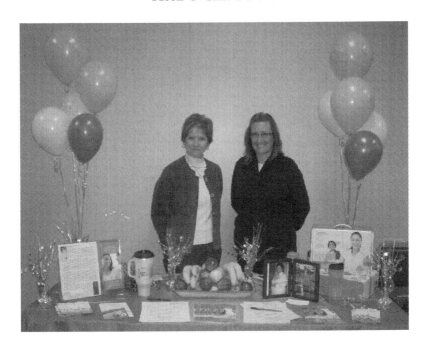

Keeli O'Cain After (with Joyce)

# Teresa Russell ~ The Detours of the Physical

My journey in First Place has been a rather long one, not because God wasn't faithful to me, but because I have not been faithful to Him. It is hard for me to admit this.

I have been overweight most of my life and my entire family is in bondage, too. We love to spend time together, and like many other families, every gathering revolves around food.

Through First Place, I learned about how God speaks to us through His Word. Our Bible study speaks to each day's situation.

In 2007, I was diagnosed with breast cancer. In October 2009, I had knee replacement surgery. More recently, I've had surgery on my ankle and ligaments. All of these surgeries are due in part to my obesity. During this time, I also lost my mother. She also suffered numerous illnesses and had numerous physical ailments due to being overweight.

When I thought being overweight was not hurting anyone, I was wrong. I hurt the ones who had to take care of me, and I stole valuable time from them. But God gave me an extended family in my First Place Bible study. God used each one to help me through my obstacles. Members covered me in prayer, laid hands on me, sent encouraging cards, and called and visited me. (God never leaves us alone.)

I know God wants me to finish the race I started more than four years ago. My advice to you is to persevere. Do not give up, even if you find yourself on a detour. It takes some of us longer than others. Everyone's journey is different.

God wants us to have healthy bodies here on earth so we can be good ambassadors of Christ. As a child of God we have received the gift of the Holy Spirit dwelling in us; therefore, we have the power within us for victory. We must die to self to receive the victory He desires for us. "So, whether we are here in this body or away from this body, our goal is to please him.

For we must all stand before Christ to be judged. We will receive whatever we deserve for the good or evil we have done in this earthly body" (2 Corinthians 5:9-10 NLT).

If physical detours slow you down and throw you off pace, don't give up. Don't quit. Get back on track. You can do this.

As of today, I have lost 50 pounds and have maintained this loss for four years. But my goal is bigger and it is time for me to move forward. My prayer is to reach my goal by the end of the year. "I press on toward the goal to win the prize for which God has called me heavenward in Christ Jesus" (Philippians 3:14 NIV).

No more detours. Persistent effort produces lasting results.

Back on track,
Teresa Russell

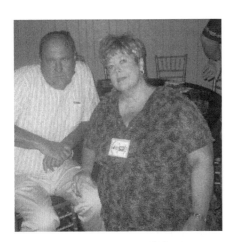

Teresa Russell Before

Teresa Russell
Back on track
(On Left)

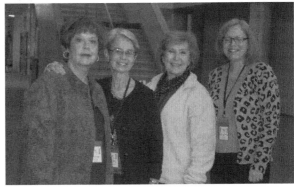

~

## Chapter 6
## Pursuing Your Promised Land ~ Run with Passion

*I pray for passion and drive now as I hit mile marker sixteen. I know I am in the place where I am about to "hit the wall." This phrase is used to describe a condition where an athlete experiences extreme fatigue due to depletion of glycogen. The question is, "Have I prepared enough?" My vision of my Promised Land, making goal weight and staying on track, letting go of every past failure or hindrance, now is the only thing that will enable me to press on and press in, and avoid hitting the wall.*

Martin Luther King Jr. will always be remembered for the words "I have a dream." He shared his dream with others. In the process, he inspired others all over this nation to reach down deep and pursue their dreams as well. Another great speech he is remembered for is the one titled "I've Been to the Mountaintop." He gave it April 3, 1968, on the eve of a protest march for striking garbage workers in Memphis, Tennessee. The next day he was assassinated. One distinctive and memorable quote in his speech helped me.

> "Well, I don't know what will happen now. We've got some difficult days ahead. But it doesn't matter with me now. Because I've been to the mountaintop. And I don't mind. Like anybody, I would like to live a long life. Longevity has its place. But I'm not concerned about that now. I just want to do God's will. And He's allowed me to go up to the mountain. And I've looked over.

And I've seen the Promised Land. I may not get there with you. But I want you to know tonight, that we, as a people, will get to the Promised Land. So I'm happy, tonight. I'm not worried about anything. I do not fear any man. Mine eyes have seen the glory of the coming of the Lord."[1]

I have had a dream, too. It has been buried deep in my heart and soul. My past failures and constant cycle of defeat for so many years caused me to remain silent in sharing my dream. Feelings of unworthiness, birthed by childhood hurts, compound my "failure mentality."

Sometimes fear of rejection or failure holds us back from sharing our dreams. Martin Luther King was a man who refused to allow fear to hold him back. He was passionate about the things he believed and that passion drove him to press on and press in, one step at a time, past every hindrance, past every encumbrance, and to see the Promised Land. His vision of, not possession of, the Promised Land encouraged him around every detour, defeat, or hindrance that might have caused him to fail.

Preparation and planning before a race, as well as pacing myself during a race, are critical for my endurance. The wall of fatigue can be seriously debilitating. Symptoms of depletion of glycogen include general weakness; fatigue; and manifestations of hypoglycemia, dizziness, and/or hallucinations. Scary information but necessary reminders to me of how important preparation, planning, training, and pacing are.

I experienced glorious days of victory as I watched the 200 mark on my scales come and go. I am now at 192 pounds with a total weight loss thus far at 137 pounds; that's a whole person. I am looking good, feeling great, and wearing a smile on my face. My high blood pressure and high cholesterol are gone.

---

[1] http://americanradioworks.publicradio.org/features/sayitplain/mlking.html

The doctor has taken me off my medications. I hear things like, "You do not want to lose too much weight and become sickly. I mean, look at how much you have already lost." You know if you hear something enough, you begin to believe that as truth. Many around me encouraged me to "just settle."

I recall a time when two and a half tribes of the Israelites decided to "just settle," too. Numbers chapter 32 tells the story of when the tribes of Ruben, Gad, and the half-tribe of Manasseh decided they wanted to live east of the Jordan River on land they had already conquered. The land was good, fertile, and fit their needs. But was it God's best? Was it God's will? God had promised them the land on the other side of the Jordan, the "Promised Land," but they were willing to settle for what they saw as good. I can so relate, because like them I have settled for less than God's very best for my life. I almost settled east of the Jordan. Settling for something good makes letting go of the dream tempting. I discovered compromise is dangerous.

Too many times, in frustration, I have settled with what I have already accomplished. But settling isn't satisfying. The sad part is seeing the scales back up on the high end and never truly finding lasting freedom from the bondage of food.

I faced the question, was I going to settle again? It would be easier than moving forward. I heard the gentle voice of Jesus say, "Don't quit; keep going." As He stirred my heart, the echo of real freedom would not let me rest or stay where I was. I was like Martin Luther King Jr. I had been to the mountaintop and I had seen the Promised Land.

As a child, I wanted others to notice me. During my teen years, I wanted to fit in, but my weight kept me in bondage and I never felt as though I measured up. I used food for comfort and security. In my marriage, I allowed food to continue to be my source of security and acceptance. In the process, I developed a problem I call closet eating.

I didn't eat much in front of others, but I did when I was alone. Eating a piece of pie was not enough; I had to eat the whole pie. A normal portion was not enough. I ate good, healthy food in front of others, but then when I was alone I consumed whole boxes of foods, eating as much as I could, until I felt sick and sluggish. I threw the empty boxes and cartons in my neighbor's trash so my husband wouldn't see them. Then I used food to reprimand myself for not living up to my potential.

I went days without eating, my punishment for poor eating habits, for making poor choices, and not sticking to my food plan. Through reward and punishment, I allowed food a place of power it was never intended to hold in my life.

I now realize this cycle fueled a failure mentality. I needed to be free. I needed to make a permanent change to break this cycle, and I was not capable of that until I acknowledged the truth. I felt like the Israelites circling in the desert, close but never quite getting to the Promised Land. Most of us don't set out to be overweight or unhealthy, but it happens. We don't intend to fall off the wagon and revert to old lifestyles and habits, but we do.

Reverting to old habits started another detour in my planned out life. I was doing well in the area of weight loss. I made time to exercise, and I ate right. I planned well and was focused, intent on making the life change really work this time. I joined a gym and started taking water aerobics. Then my husband's dad died and his mom, in the early stages of Alzheimer's, came to live with us.

My world and my plans were turned upside-down. My husband and I owned a high-stress business, and now we added around-the-clock supervision of his mother, all while grieving the loss of his father. The chaos and emotional stress of going from a planned and controlled household to an extra housemate with multiple sitters and family coming and going like it was Grand Central Station was too much for me to handle.

I gave up my time at the gym. My life and my plans were no longer mine. My schedule revolved around my husband's mom. Research shows caregivers are affected most in cases of Alzheimer patients. I believed it, because I was experiencing it. Nothing in my life felt normal. The more I tried to control things the more out of control they got. My emotional roller coaster picked up speed.

At one of its steepest points, my roller coaster came careening down the track with amazing speed, landing in the middle of a blueberry cream cheese pie. My husband loves my cooking and I love cooking for him. (When we met, I made the terrible mistake of cooking a meal for him and never could get rid of him afterwards.) I tell him he fell in love with my cooking before he fell in love with me.

One of Glenn's favorite food items is blueberry cream cheese pie, with my special homemade crust made with pastry flour, butter, and pecans. I agreed to make it for him one day. I put the final touches on the pie topping and placed it in the refrigerator. While the pie was chilling, I tended to Glenn's mother. Suddenly, she passed out in my arms. Glenn and I feared she was dead, but with quick-thinking paramedics and a speedy ambulance ride, she was admitted to the hospital for tests.

Glenn sat with his mother at the hospital. I was home alone— with the pie. I ate one piece, but I didn't stop at one piece. I ate three. With each bite, I blamed myself. How was I going to explain to Glenn that I had eaten half a pie? I decided to finish it off. Destroy the evidence. With the traumatic events of the day, Glenn would never remember asking me to make it for him.

Several weeks went by and my old cycle was back in place. Food once again had a hold on me. I was miserable, but I couldn't seem to do anything about it. I was so far down in the pit. I didn't think I could pull myself out.

I called a dear friend, confiding in her the events that had caused me to stumble in the process of my journey. With God's grace, I reached past the shame and guilt and cried for help. The Lord provided the right person to help me climb from my imprisoning pit.

The Word of God is filled with promises. Until we possess these promises, they are nothing more than words in a book. "Possess" is an active verb meaning "to take hold of." If I was going to reach out for everything He promised, I needed to be active and believe God.

God did not only want to change my body shape and size. He wanted to do a complete recovery of my whole person, if I would allow Him to do it. I finally and fully trusted God for the outcome of my journey.

With God in control, there is no turning back. No more settling for less than goal. I was headed to the finish line. Faith is not believing in spite of evidence but obeying in spite of consequence. The Lord wanted me to choose life. With God's help, I could achieve my short-term and long-term goals. My success would not be built on my strength but His power.

Every day we are faced with choices, and God allows us to choose. Remember, choices bring either blessings or curses (life or death). Doing my part was (and still is) a daily process. The pathway to success would lead to a glorious destination if I was willing to choose to walk with God, learning to enjoy the journey in getting there.

The Lord built a fire in my heart, a fire that became a blazing flame. I chose to acknowledge the reasons for past failures and work through the emotions that caused the derailment of my good intentions. I was committed this time to building a team of accountability around me and I purposed never to go back to the other side of 200 pounds.

Settling for less than His best is not acceptable. I choose, like Martin Luther King Jr., not to allow fear to keep me from real and lasting freedom.

I never want to give up again. Success is not by accident. I choose to remain on the path. I must follow to completion. I stopped looking at what I was being freed from and focused on what I was being "freed to."

I was being freed to love God; to achieve a healthy goal weight; and to live in His fullness, under His protection, and with His provision. I wanted to allow the Lord to complete the good work He began in me. I finally understood that knowing God and reflecting His glory is the true pathway to success.

God warned me there would be giants in the Promised Land. Giants must be defeated for me to take possession of my new lifestyle. The one holding me in His hands is able to defeat any giants on my behalf. I must continue to do my part, but from my new vantage point I feel anything is finally possible, even the defeat of giants. I sense in my spirit that there will be other detours, higher hills, deeper valleys, twists and turns, and possibly future desert wanderings. I will have to draw upon my faith to keep going, but I am stepping into the swirling waters of the Jordan. I can see the Promise Land.

I want to be like Martin Luther King Jr. and like Moses. They both went to the mountaintop and saw their Promised Land. It was enough for them, and it is enough for me, too.

Life change costs something. I'm facing a wall now, a serious stage. I only have a few more pounds left to lose. Those last pounds are like the last miles in a race. Will I quit or will I put one foot in front of the other? I am close to the final barrier between the finish line and me.

I decide to focus on my rhythm and fight the doubts. I am trusting in the training and preparation and I believe I am prepared for what is ahead. The fuel from my spiritual, emotional, mental, and physical reserves give me confidence, one stride after the other and one mile at a time. These last ten pounds really seem impossible, but I am determined to finish. Will I make it this time? Yes, because the days I cannot run I will walk by faith.

## * Personal Reflection:  Focus on Life Change

We all face daily challenges. How we perceive a challenge is integral in how we solve the problem. When we are overwhelmed or find it difficult to overcome, we must dig down deep, focus on the prize or the goal, and keep taking one step at a time. When progress seems slow, don't stop.

Some challenges will be physical, some mental, some emotional, and some will be spiritual. We can overcome all obstacles and achieve our goals if we passionately pursue the Promised Land. Only then will we experience real freedom and life change.

Pursuing balance is an ongoing process, and charting your progress is meant to keep you on track. Exercise discipline and eliminate bad habits and poor excuses, and you will overcome pitfalls. Take baby steps in making changes.

Moving forward regardless of my pace allows me to understand how God weaves life events, including my past and present pain, into a glorious tapestry. Making it through a physical race or a life race takes confidence and resolve. Some days the desire to quit seems overwhelming. Keep taking the next step forward. Put one foot in front of the other. When you cannot run, resolve to walk by faith.

Ask God to show you the dream He has for you. Learn to establish some short- and long-term goals in relation to success. Be aware of difficulties and be willing to ask for help, but don't be afraid to dream. Dream big.

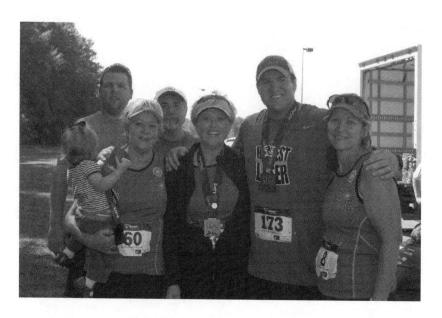

Half-Marathon – With Patrick House of *The Biggest Loser* TV show

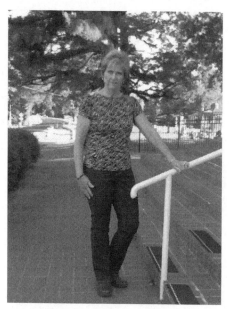

~ Joyce ~

# Chapter 7
## Taking Possession ~ Removing the Final Barriers

*Why am I running this race? I want to stop. The fatigue is a wall. But I have come too far to turn around. Going back or quitting are no longer options. I can only go forward. Doubt and exhaustion nibble at my resolve. As I struggle to finish I need to be mentally and emotionally tough. I must dig deep.*

*I made it this far because of planning, preparation, and training. And good advice and assistance from others helped get me here, too. Experienced marathoners, running books and magazines, life coaches, friends that trained and ran with me, and store clerks knowledgeable in training gear have helped me along my way. Can I get past this next barrier?*

Seeking sound counsel and trustworthy advice helps motivate us, but at some point, we have to do more. We have to keep going. We have to take the advice and apply it. Do you have as much trouble convincing yourself of this as I do? Fear can hold us back.

I can train for all sorts of races, but if I don't register, show up, and actually run I have still only trained, never tested my training. The same is true for weight loss and for life. We can get help, good advice, and knowledge, but if we never make changes and get into the race, all our knowledge is for naught. The purpose of training is to prepare us to run not prepare us to remain still.

In Joshua 3:5, Joshua told the people to consecrate themselves because the Lord was about to do mighty things. As the children of Israel stood on the banks of the Jordan River, they prepared to enter the Promised Land. One day, I stood at the banks of my Jordan River, and the Lord was about to teach me lessons in trust and obedience.

The banks of the Jordan are a faith-building place. There I will surrender completely to God or I will never get my feet wet. My faith-building place started in my doctor's office for my yearly check-up. I really loved going, getting test results and profiles checked. With my weight in the 170-pound range, I didn't mind getting on the scales anymore. What I hated was having blood drawn and the actual exam. My doctor commended me for my good work. He encouraged me about my weight loss and we talked about my continued effort toward goal weight.

During my exam, he gently grasped a double handful of loose skin and said that I really needed to consider having the excess skin removed. He said, "Removing this skin will make you look and feel better."

I joked, "The skin is mine, kinda like a good friend, and I think I'll keep it as long as the fat that was once inside it never returns."

My sweet doctor, who had seen me through so much, looked deeply into my eyes and said, "You know, maybe it is time to remove the final barrier between you and lasting freedom from the weight you have lost. You are choosing to continue to carry excess baggage that is not necessary or needed any longer. Why are you choosing to hang on to it when you can be free from it?"

I gave no answer and determined to put his probing question out of my mind. As I left his office he again praised my success, and then patted my arm. "I hope you'll reconsider seeing a doctor about having the excess skin removed." I smiled one last time and said I would give it some thought. I didn't intend to consider it. I had a terrible fear of needles, blood, and hospitals. I know this sounds crazy, but I had my first child by natural childbirth just because I did not want to have a shot. Now, that's fear of needles!

Had the surgery been necessary I would have dealt with it, but to willingly decide to have myself put in a hospital, let someone cut on me, and put a needle in my arm, well, it was just not happening. Or so I thought.

Over the next couple of months I tried to put the doctor's suggestion out of my mind. I refused to consider the procedure. I refused to consider having the excess skin removed, and I refused to try to answer my doctor's probing questions. I was willing to settle (there's that word again) for the way I was. And in addition to my fear of hospitals, blood, and needles, I also feared what other people would say.

I continued to make slow progress toward my weight-loss goal. Each pound lost seemed harder to attain, but at least I was still headed in the right direction. Life became more balanced. I taught a FP4H class and I had a great team of accountability partners that helped me stay on track and focused. My husband and I sold our business at a healthy profit; the years of hard work and dedication had paid off.

We decided to travel. So we visited the Holy Land and Alaska. When we returned, we each took a job just to continue to work, but in less stressful environments than running our own company had been. These changes allowed us more free time to focus on making lasting and positive changes in our lifestyle, as well as volunteering in our church and community.

There were times, however, when I was dressing for work or church that I grabbed the excess skin and wondered about what my doctor had recommended. What would it be like to have it removed? Even though I wore smaller clothes than before, the excess skin took up a lot of space and I had to buy clothes and undergarments larger than I should have just to accommodate the surplus skin. Some of my undergarments were expensive because of the extra support and functionality they provided.

It reminded me of having an apron on all the time. At the beginning of my journey, I had not considered the fact that I would have excess skin or that it would be a problem. I only focused on the weight loss.

I foolishly thought that the skin expanded to accommodate the excess weight as I put the weight on and it would tighten back up after the weight was gone. I had never lost this much weight before and had never dealt with the problem.

The thought of having the skin removed was scary, but there was a deeper issue. Why was I so against having the excess skin removed? In some ways, I felt that the excess skin was my punishment for all the years of abuse I had given my body. It was as if this was my cross and I should bear it. There, I said it.

My cross was a load of guilt for one person to carry; in fact it probably weighed more than the skin. Still, I pushed the thoughts away again, one more time refusing to process the truth, not quite ready to face the guilt or fear that held me back.

Like mile markers in a race as you near the finish line, reality in dealing with my excess skin came my way faster than I expected. In December I experienced some health issues. Up to this point, I was the healthiest I had been in years.

My doctor thought I had a hormonal imbalance from all the weight loss, and then thought my problems were pre-menopausal. I thought I was having a break down. I cried all the time, experienced night sweats, a racing heart, soaking wet clothes, and severe lower abdominal pain. This went on for a short time and after extensive testing, my doctor finally realized I had a cyst on one of my ovaries. Because of the high risk of ovarian cancer for women my age it did not appear I had a lot of options. The best option, according to my doctor, was an oophorectomy. I needed to have my ovaries removed.

As my doctor and I discussed the surgery options he said, "There will never be a better time to get that skin removed than now. You have to have surgery anyway. I want to refer you to a plastic surgeon; it will be the best thing you will ever choose to do for yourself besides losing all that weight. Having the skin removed is a wise decision for you to consider." He continued, "This is not about looking better, it is about taking the best care of your body."

In my mind the barriers between me and having this skin removed were still too many. How did I get myself into this? At this point, having the skin removed was still not something I considered necessary, but now I was willing to consider the option, if for no other reason than to make my doctor feel better. I asked more questions. He talked. I listened. And finally I agreed to see the plastic surgeon. Whatever the answer, there was only one thing to do. Keep going.

I did not have a positive experience with the first plastic surgeon. My husband went with me for the appointment. We prayed before we went into the office asking the Lord for his direction and wisdom. The doctor did not spend a lot of personal time answering our questions. I left his office unsure and disappointed with the whole process. We decided he was not the doctor for us and I decided that this surgery might possibly not be for me.

However, God had another plan. Earlier that year I'd had some problems with one of my hands and my doctor referred me to a hand specialist, but I'd never made a follow-up appointment with him. Just as I was ready to decide against the plastic surgery a friend who is a nurse told me about a surgeon who had done a procedure for her and how very pleased she was with the quality of his work. She said he was a board certified plastic and cosmetic surgeon. He turned out to be the same doctor I had been referred to for my hand. I believed it was God's confirmation in leading me to the correct surgeon.

The time for my oophorectomy surgery was fast approaching, so I decided to call and set up a consultation with the plastic surgeon. Might as well, I needed someone to look at my hand anyway. A few days later I met with Dr. Kenneth R. Barraza, a plastic and reconstructive surgeon certified by the American Board of Plastic Surgery. This doctor came highly recommended by several trusted individuals, but the real test was about to happen.

My first impression was of a trusted friend. He presented himself as a professional deeply concerned with patient care, which at this moment happened to be me. He allowed me to ask questions and he gave answers in a thoughtful and sincere way. He examined the excess skin. We discussed the procedures and the risks. We talked about my weight-loss journey, my general health, the impact surgery has on a spouse, and what to expect before and after surgery.

Next, I had a discussion with Dr. Barraza's assistant about procedure cost and recovery time. They were both helpful and allowed me to ask all the questions that plagued me about this process. That day I realized how important doctor selection is for something this important and costly. I left feeling at peace with all the information I had obtained.

Talking to someone you know and trust is another important part of the process of making choices. I called my friend for advice and reassurance.

My friend and her husband not only talked with us but invited us to their home and allowed my husband and me to ask all the questions we wanted to ask. They shared openly with us, even down to how the spouse felt before and after the surgery and how it had affected their relationship. This dear friend shared the emotional life change she experienced through this procedure. She said the surgery was one of the best things she had ever done for herself and she had no regrets. The surgery changed her outlook on life.

I began to see that this was more than just a skin removal process in the physical sense, but also a natural and needed part of the journey to real freedom. I am forever thankful for friends who were willing to open up their home, give us their time, and openly and honestly share their lives.

I worried that having this surgery done could be considered vain. I didn't want to be considered vain by my Lord. I decided my next stop would be for spiritual counsel. Having this surgery was not a decision I was willing to enter into lightly. I needed all the facts prior to surgery.

The next few weeks were quite a journey for us. We met with a trusted Christian counselor, met again with Dr. Barraza, and had an additional in-depth discussion on the procedures. We learned how one procedure would complement the other and about the cost savings in having the recommended procedures done at the same time. We discussed recovery time and care needed afterwards. The cost for this type of surgery can be expensive, and insurance rarely pays for it. This was probably the greatest barrier we had to scale in the whole decision-making process. How do you put a price tag on this? We prayed, we talked, we prayed, and talked some more. And through all this decision-making, my husband and I found a new place in our marriage.

We became closer than we had ever been before. He was so supportive, understanding, and loving, and we walked hand in hand through this mile marker, still focusing on the finish. My journey greatly affected my husband who had married a woman who weighed almost 300 pounds some seventeen years earlier. He had seen and been part of a lot of change over the last few years. I was less than half the woman I use to be. Literally.

He is my best friend and did not let me down in this leg of the race. He stood beside me, encouraged me to have the surgery, asked questions, helped gather facts, and prayed with me and for me. It was his encouragement, the confidence in our doctor, and faith that the Lord had provided the right surgeon for us that gave me the peace I needed to finally agree to the procedure.

"Let's do it."

I was still afraid of the unknown but trusted in my Savior to see me through. The battle in my mind and heart had been fought and won, and in that space was a sense of peace. It was time to take the next step.

Remember the initial question my doctor had asked? Why did I choose to hang on to something that I could be freed from? The idea moved to the forefront of my thought process. Was there something deeper here than I realized? Removing the excess skin in a sense for me was a sign of surrender of the whole person to this new life. It was as if to say, "I am never going back. I am stepping past the final barrier between the new life and the old. There will be nothing to go back to. It is gone. It has been removed."

I learned that God is not in the business of punishment. He is the God of restoration. His desire has always been and will always be to restore us unto Himself. His desire was a total and complete healing in my life. I finally realized that He wants me to be a whole person spiritually, mentally, physically, and emotionally. He holds nothing back. I was at the final barrier. It was time to find my second wind. The finish line was just ahead.

A week after Mother's Day in a small private hospital, I stepped past that physical barrier of excess skin into a new place in my life. Along with the needed bilateral oophorectomy surgery, I also had a bilateral mastopexy, which is a breast lift. The procedure raised and firmed the breasts by removing excess skin and tightening the surrounding tissue to reshape and support the new breast contour. The final procedure was a belt lipectomy, or body lift, which removed the excess skin from hip to hip in the front and extended all the way around to the back. It tightened the underlying abdominal muscles and lifted the thighs and buttocks by removing all the excess skin in those areas.

My incision extended all the way around to the spine. I jokingly tell my husband I have been cut in half and sewn back together. There was a lot going on in that operating room. Eight hours later I made an entrance in recovery. The next day I went home under the care of my beloved husband and a few close friends. I had made it through the physical barrier of the skin removal process, but the emotional barrier that I had to face was still ahead. The words life-changing were about to take on a whole new meaning for me.

# * Personal Reflection: Discover the Freedom

The process of skin removal surgery was a daunting process for me personally. Doctor selection, an understanding of the procedures needed, all those factors were important, including how much weight I had lost, how much loose skin I had, cost, recovery time, and seeking answers to the spiritual questions. All those components were significant. Peace with my decision was critical. I am a private and sensitive person. Seeking out wisdom and direction for this procedure caused me to step past my comfort zone.

My advice is to be willing to step out of your comfort zone, if that is what it takes to get the answers you need. Know your options. Know your options for your physical, emotional, and spiritual health.

My total out-of-pocket cost for the combination of the three procedures was a little over $16,000. If I'd had the skin removal surgery done separately from the bilateral oophorectomy, my out-of-pocket cost would have been more. Prices vary from doctor to doctor and from area to area. Most doctors have set fees for certain procedures, but there are many variable costs involved that have to be considered. The key component for me was not the cost as much as the doctor selection, and following God's direction.

The surgery is by far the best thing I have ever done for myself apart from losing the weight and surrendering to the Lord. I am thankful for a husband who was supportive and willing to sacrifice financially. The surgery brought with it the most emotionally healing aspects of my weight-loss journey. It allowed me to find answers to questions I had from years of yo-yo dieting. I had played that losing and gaining game far too long.

The surgery allowed me to step into a new-found freedom from the emotional bondage of food. The skin removal process has given me additional determination to never go back to the bondage of food. After my substantial weight loss the skin removal surgery gave me the completed results I needed. It was the final barrier that I needed removed from my life.

My journey has made my marriage stronger and my faith deeper. The only thing I regret about my surgery is not discussing it beforehand with my adult children. I now realize that deciding to wait until after the surgery to share my decision with them was not wise on my part. It scared my kids to death. Sorry, kids. Mom's not perfect.

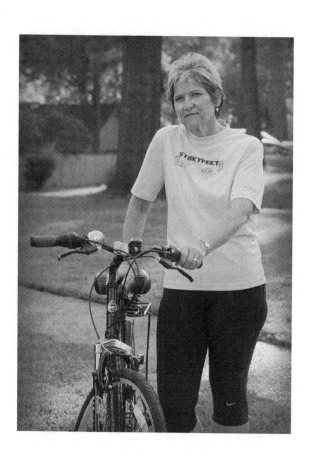

# Question and Answer with Kenneth R. Barraza, M.D.

I believe without a doubt that the Lord led me through a series of events to Dr. Kenneth Barraza. He is the physician who performed my surgical procedures. Dr. Barraza is a plastic and reconstructive surgeon certified by the American Board of Plastic Surgery. He has 20 years of experience performing all types of plastic and reconstructive procedures including those associated with massive weight loss. He maintains a busy practice in Jackson, Mississippi.

Asking questions and seeking answers is the only way to get facts. The following questions are those that several individuals including myself have asked about surgical procedures related to weight loss. Dr. Barraza graciously consented to answer these questions. I hope the answers will enable others to make an informed decision about whether surgery is right for them.

Q: Dr. Barraza, what can you tell us in general about excessive amounts of skin due to weight loss?

A: Many people who have achieved significant weight loss can be left with large amounts of heavy, loose skin around the abdomen, back, buttocks, breasts, thighs, arms, and face. The skin may lose elasticity and sag as a result of being stretched for long periods of time. It often fails to shrink back to its former size and shape after weight loss. Some consider this skin excess a cosmetic issue. However, in many instances it can cause health and hygiene issues such as rashes, sores, and infections. Yeast infections under skin folds are very common, which can result in foul odor and irritation. The sheer weight of the hanging skin excess may cause back pain. Not only physical but also emotional and social issues may result. Those who have lost a large amount of weight and who are committed to a new lifestyle want their bodies to reflect a new, more positive image. The only way to remove this excess and help alleviate these problems is through plastic surgical procedures.

Q: What criteria do you look for when determining if a patient is a good candidate for having skin removal surgery?

A: Generally, good health is the most important criteria. Patients should be free from heart and lung disease, diabetes, and other major medical problems. Their weight should be stable and good nutritional habits should be in place. Smokers are not considered candidates unless they are able to quit smoking completely. Smoking increases the risk of serious complications both during and after surgery. A good candidate should be mentally and emotionally stable. Patients must have realistic expectations. Surgery will lead to marked improvements in body shape, but it is impossible to restore the body to what it would have been without the weight gain.

Q: So can a person have all the skin excess removed at the same time with one surgery?

A: In most cases, no. A combination of procedures may be done at the same time as long as safety can be maintained, but in most cases multiple stages will be needed. Skin reduction is done in stages to minimize complications such as blood loss or blood clots. It is often done over an extended period of time addressing one or two areas per stage. The surgeon should make recommendations about the best strategy to address all of his patients' specific needs in the safest and most efficient manner.

Q: Can you give us an idea of some of the procedures that might be considered for excess skin removal?

A: There are a number of procedures that one could consider. In most cases your surgeon will work with you to identify areas that are the most problematic or bothersome to you and advise you as to which procedure or procedures you would qualify for as a candidate. These are the areas of the body most often addressed:

*Abdomen: Abdominoplasty, also known as a "tummy tuck," involves removing excess skin of the abdomen and tightening of the underlying muscles. An incision is made just above the pubic area from hip to hip. Sometimes a vertical incision is necessary. Panniculectomy is simply the removal of excess skin without muscle repair. This may be indicated in some patients.

*Buttocks/upper thighs: Belt-lipectomy, also known, as a "body lift," is the most common and essential procedure for weight-loss patients. It is an abdominoplasty, which is extended to include the back and buttocks areas. This allows for removal of skin excess as well as lifting and tightening of the outer thigh and buttocks. The resulting scar is circumferential around the lower trunk.

*Thighs: The medial thigh-lift removes excess skin and lifts and tightens the upper inner thigh area.

*Breasts: A number of breast-related procedures are available including breast lift (mastopexy) with or without augmentation (implants) and breast reduction. These procedures lift and tighten the breast by removing excess skin to restore breast shape and contour. Implants may be necessary not for size but for shape and contour.

*Arms: Brachioplasty removes excess skin from the arm. An incision is made starting at the armpit and extending to the elbow.

*Face and neck: Removing excessive skin of the face and neck after weight loss is similar to a traditional neck lift or face lift. Resulting scars are not perceptible as incisions are strategically planned in front of the ear and along the hairline.

A typical sequence of staged procedures would be:

1) Belt-lipectomy plus breast surgery
2) Medial thigh lift plus brachioplasty
3) Neck lift or face lift

Not all patients will need or choose to have all of the procedures or stages. The stage 1 procedures are most commonly done.

Q: What can I expect to happen on my first visit?

A: During an initial consultation, I normally perform a careful history and physical examination. I assess the individual's physical and emotional health and discuss specific goals for the surgery. We then openly discuss expectations to make certain that they are in line with what can be realistically expected from the procedure. I can then determine the best plan for you. I explain details of the procedure, its potential risks and complications, as well as the recovery experience. We also discuss cost as well as where the procedure will be performed and the length of stay.

Q: What things should an individual consider before having skin removal surgery?

A: The most important factor to me is stability of weight. Equally important is that my patients are close to their weight-loss goal. Surgery is not a substitute for further weight loss nor will it be a motivation to maintain your dietary habits and exercise regimen. Patients should be of good health physically, nutritionally, and emotionally. They should have realistic expectations and these should be discussed with the doctor.

Q: Are there risks associated with skin removal procedures?

A: Any surgical procedure carries some risk although these risks are usually minimal in the well-selected patient. Resulting scars can be significant. Infection or bleeding (hematoma) is possible as are fluid collections (seroma). Blood clots that could lead to pulmonary embolism are fortunately rare. Touchup or revision procedures are occasionally necessary.

Q: What do I expect during the time around surgery?

A: In many cases these procedures are performed on an outpatient basis in an outpatient surgical facility. Some may require hospitalization with a one- or two-night stay. Surgical drains are typically placed and will remain for about five days. Medications are given to control pain and discomfort.

Q: How long is the normal recovery time?

A: Recovery time is fairly rapid but is highly patient dependent. Typically I would expect a return to work in about two weeks. Full activity including vigorous exercise routines could resume in about four to six weeks. The first seventy-two hours after surgery are the most uncomfortable It is extremely important to begin ambulation the first day postoperatively. Remaining motionless in the bed is a setup for blood clots. Pain medicine is supplied and is important during this initial period.

Q: Will my insurance pay for any of these procedures?

A: Currently, most insurance companies do not cover procedures related to removal of skin excess after massive weight loss. Complications that might result are likewise generally not covered. There are a few ancillary procedures that might be considered for insurance coverage. For instance, a hernia repair or a scar revision related to previous covered surgical procedures.

Q: What is the cost associated with skin removal surgeries?

A: The cost of skin removal surgery varies from clinic to clinic and from one region of the country to another. The surgeon's fee is based on the number of procedures performed at each stage. In addition to the surgeon's fee there are fees for anesthesia and for the surgical facility. Specific fees are itemized at the time of the initial consultation. Financial coordinators are available to discuss payment options.

Q: Are there any nonsurgical procedures with a similar outcome for individuals with skin excess following massive weight loss.

A: No.

Q: What about the emotional aspects of having this type of surgery?

A: Achieving our goal for these patients requires a process that can consist of multiple stages over a prolonged time period. It is extremely important that patients are prepared emotionally for that process. Having a realistic expectation for results is crucial. The surgery can impact not only the patient but also the spouse and the entire family. This should be considered preoperatively. The end result of this process, however, can be remarkable. I don't believe I've ever had a patient that regretted having gone through the process. They often feel as though their life has been given back to them. They typically have renewed self-esteem and improved outlook. For most it is the completion of the entire weight-loss process.

Q: Can you provide details from my surgical consultation? (Joyce Ainsworth)

A: After our initial consultation I felt as though you were an excellent candidate for multiple procedures related to your weight loss. You were found to be healthy, fit, and emotionally prepared. You were found to have extreme skin excess and laxity throughout the abdominal and back areas as well as the thighs, arms, and breast areas. You had laxity and separation of the abdominal muscles. Your skin tone was poor and with a lot of surface irregularity. My recommendation was for a belt-lipectomy and bilateral mastopexy (breast lift).These procedures were planned in conjunction with an oophorectomy to be done by your gynecologist. Brachioplasty and medial thigh lift were possibilities for a second stage.

The surgery was done as an overnight stay in the hospital (due to the combined gynecologic procedure). Surgery lasted approximately eight hours. There were no complications. The drains were removed during the first postoperative visit at about one week. Your final follow-up was at six weeks postoperatively. You have an excellent result and you certainly seem to be very pleased.

Q: Is there any advice you would give someone who is considering this type of surgery?

A: Losing a large amount of weight is a major accomplishment that will enhance your health, your appearance, and your outlook on life. Get the facts and see if skin removal surgery is an option for you. Make certain your weight-loss goal has been met and you are sound physically and emotionally.

Do not expect measurable weight loss after these procedures, although it will likely result eventually. Most patients will note that the time and expense associated with this surgery is well spent toward the completion of their journey to better physical and emotional health.

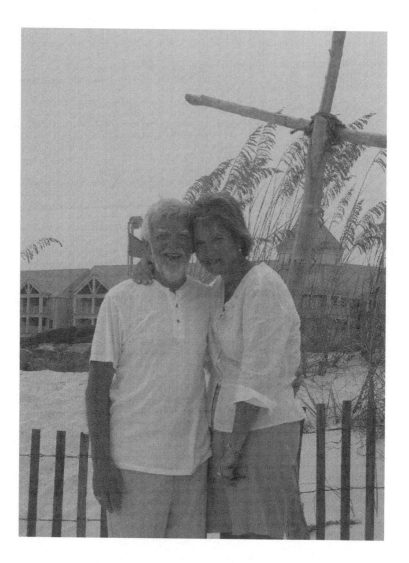

Joyce and Glenn Ainsworth

~

# Chapter 8
## The Second Wind ~ Find New Strength

*I am exhausted and I begin to think about quitting. I rationalize, "I've made it farther than ever before. Won't everyone be proud of what I've done so far? I'm at mile marker twenty. Isn't it enough? I could drop out now and no one would think badly of me." Then something amazing happens. Fresh, new breath. A second wind. It feels as if my feet are flying. My shoes feel lighter. I push forward. I have new strength. I'm running faster and freer than ever. I can almost see it. The finish line. Not much farther now. I can do it. I am stronger than ever.*

Runners often talk about a point when they feel too exhausted to continue. Instead of slowing dramatically or quitting, these runners continue to run at a strong pace and often exceed their personal expectations. Some call this surge in energy a "second wind," while others call it "new-found strength." Studies show and some scientists believe this strange phenomenon occurs when the runner's body finds enough oxygen to counteract the buildup of lactic acid in the muscles. Others think the second wind experience is a result of endorphin production, like a runner's high. I believe the feeling is psychological, an attitude adjustment and a surge of confidence happens. I also think a second wind can occur as the runner hears strong encouragement from spectators and other runners.

Having my excess skin removed was like finding a second wind for me. It was a deep breath of confidence and energy. And a freedom I can't explain. Three weeks after surgery I started walking again and by my six-week check-up I walked three miles a day. It was as if my feet had wings and I could walk as never before.

Recovery was not yet complete, but I was headed in the right direction. Don't think this made the final pounds of my weight-loss goal any faster or any easier. I was still in the high 150-pound weight range and I knew I had not reached my finish line.

I had lugged the excessive skin around for a while, as though I carried an extra package or backpack all the time. My excessive weight of skin was not only a physical burden; it was a mental, emotional, and spiritual burden. Once it was removed, I felt odd without my familiar cargo. I had grown accustomed to the weight, and I really noticed the difference when I started walking and running again. I seemed to be floating and couldn't remember a time I felt so light. The result was buoyancy. Walking and running never felt so good. I understood what Paul meant in Scripture when he said to strip off every weight that slows us down, or hinders us, especially the sin that so easily trips us up. I could now enjoy exercise, like running and walking, and be more successful at doing these activities than ever before.

My newfound strength helped me press forward into the final stretch of my journey. It gave me renewed energy, self-esteem, and confidence. I had learned to love exercise, but now loving exercise has a new meaning for me. I not only love to walk/run, but I enjoy working out in the gym. I love to take classes like body pump, yogilates, and water aerobics. I now have the courage and strength to become the best I can be. If exercise is going to be a part of the rest of my life, and it really has to be, then I need to keep it fun, challenging, exciting, and interesting.

I am determined to continue stepping out of my comfort zone and trying new things. I experiment with new exercises, keep the ones I enjoy, and sideline the ones I don't. I am challenged by new, different, and exciting exercises. My new nickname is "Gym Junkie." I suppose if I am going to be a junkie, a gym junkie isn't a bad kind of junkie to be. I tell myself that I love exercise, I love exercise, I love exercise.

I speak positive affirmations and truths into my life. I want my journey to have a different long-term mental outcome than in the past. I never want to go back to the bondage of food or to excessive weight -- not ever again. Okay, so my mind is there. What's next?

Having the issue settled in my mind was not the final and total transformation I needed. I would need to go at least one step further. My next obstacle was to change my deepest desire so that I would never want to go back. If my desire to be bondage-free was stronger than the allure of food, then I would be successful. In the past, I had wanted a long-term solution but never surrendered my actions to a new way of life. As I pondered the idea of desire and action change, the word "action" jumped out at me.

In the past, I had a short-term mindset. Losing weight was great. Fitting into smaller sizes was fun. The new energy was wonderful. Even my hope to stay fit and healthy was good, but something had to happen to ensure I would never want to go back. The Lord began to show me how my actions had to change. My intentions and motives wouldn't carry me into the future. I needed to change my actions. And be willing to sacrifice my desires until I no longer wanted to go back. The same dependence on Him I developed getting here was what He wanted me to learn to live by, not sometimes or for a season, but daily and every day for a lifetime.

Changing my actions became my newfound strength. I realized real life change happened in the journey to the finish line, not at the finish line or because of the finish line. The first time I saw myself in a mirror after I was healed from the surgery and free from my excessive skin, I wept. I broke down and cried like a baby because, for the first time since my journey began, I saw a new person emerging. The surgery had stripped away my skin and along with it my ugly barriers and all the accompanying fears, frustrations, and failures.

The chains of bondage were broken and for the first time I experienced a joy from deep inside that overflowed as if from a well-spring within me, bubbling up as if uncontainable. I saw the beauty of Jesus revealed in me. In me! How humbling. I had been a Christian before my weight loss, but now the beauty of Jesus' reflection glowed in a new and different way.

Here was beauty and change. Then I saw the green eyes of this new woman staring back at me. As I gazed into those beautiful green eyes, I no longer saw a stranger but a free woman.

For way too long I felt my weight and excess skin were punishment for years of poor choices and abuse I gave my body. Guilt had been my constant companion. I believed being overweight was my cross to bear, and I deserved to bear it. I built guilt into my personality. In the past, I had tried to lose weight and get healthy with a failure mentality, which allowed me only a small level of success before I defaulted back to my old patterns. A never-ending cycle of hope, guilt, and failure happened repeatedly and every new poor choice or failure added to the pile of debris. Once I allowed the guilt to control, losing hope had always been the next step. No wonder I did not know who I was or could not imagine the person I could become.

I wonder how many of us feel burdened by false guilt. We never say it aloud, but it is there etched deep in our hearts and subconscious minds. Only the healing power of Christ can touch this place in each of us. A load of false guilt and hopelessness is too much for one person to carry. I unloaded the heavy weight in front of the mirror that day. I realized my guilt weighed more than the skin the doctor removed. No wonder I felt light and free.

Discovering the spiritual aspect of my journey is my new-found-strength. One more chain fell off and God did a new spiritual work in my life. Now I refuse to push the thoughts of freedom away, and God has liberated me from the lies of Satan.

One of the names of God found in the Old Testament is El Roi. The name means "the God who sees me." Hagar used this name in Genesis 16:13. She ran away in despair and fear. But God saw her. I finally realized God has seen my afflictions and He loves me anyway. He loved me as I was and orchestrated a plan of healing that surpassed the issue of weight in my life. God's desire is and always will be to restore us unto Him.

The path to my freedom started when I walked into a FP4H class with the mindset that this was my last hope. Recovery and restoration began in my life that day. I am thankful that I not only have a God who saw my afflictions (El Roi) but also the Lord who heals (Jehovah-Rapha).

My restoration is a journey from unhealthy to strong, from overweight to beauty deeper than my skin. Physical beauty is one thing, spiritual beauty is life changing. God's work will continue until my journey ends in heaven.

After my surgery, a dear friend gave me a list of positive affirmations and encouraged me to say them aloud to myself every day. These affirmations were based on truths in God's Word. Wounded people like me cannot understand the power of the spoken word until we see the healing that comes from speaking "truth" into our lives.

I clearly recall the first time I spoke those affirmations aloud. I felt silly and Satan tried to convince me these pronouncements were not true, but as days passed into weeks, I heard the words and I felt them filter from my ears to my heart. Once again the dam broke and a flood of healing tears washed over my life. The words felt like salve applied to a deep, gaping wound, a wound that had festered for a long time and was now beginning to heal. My spoken affirmations were life changing. I continue using those positive affirmations in my life daily.

Why? It takes time to uproot and replace the hurts, hang-ups, and untruths.

In the appendix, you will find a copy of the positive affirmations I continue to use daily. These affirmations are simply examples. You can create a list for yourself and make them personal for you or make the list I share your own.

I had new-found strength from the skin reduction surgery and I had taken the first steps toward spiritual healing by allowing God to change my desires. I conquered relying on food as my comfort and friend. But I faced one larger hurdle - my pride.

In the past when I lost weight I loved the attention and acceptance I received from friends and acquaintances. Then some life event such as a tragedy or sickness or even a party gave me an excuse to return to my bad food habits. I justified the behavior because I felt so good about myself and it seemed others liked me, too. Eating unhealthy snacks and meals was more than making wrong food choices. I descended into a spiritual breakdown, losing sight of God's power in my life and reaffirming my undeserving and unworthy self-judgment. Emotionally, I defaulted to food again instead of turning to the Lord and allowing Christ to show me the truth that could really set me free.

I now realize the life change had not been complete in those other dieting experiences. For so many years I had been a yo-yo dieter, playing a losing and gaining game. Lose a little. Feel good about it. Gain it back (and more). This time I won't stop until I reach the finish line – my goal weight. This time I won't stop at partial success. The final hurdle is behind me now. The weight loss I've experienced has nothing to do with a scale.

When the children of Israel traveled toward the Promised Land, they laid memorial stones in places where God had shown up to rescue the nation. I decided to begin placing memorial stones as I move forward. Each stone reminds me of my life change process. I placed a stone where I started at 339 pounds. I want to remember where I've come from and I purpose in my heart never to return to the other side of the Jordan. I've placed a stone in front of my mirror. I always want to remember the truly precious, vitally important, and historic change that took place in my heart that day.

The journey to life change is long and hard. It has not been easy by any stretch of the imagination. God did not take the Israelites on the shortest route to the Promised Land either. The forty-year journey through the wilderness taught them who He was. There were daily battles and giants to defeat as they learned to depend totally on Him. Through my physical battles and emotional and spiritual healing, I am ready for the finish line, too.

What now? I stepped on the scales this morning. My weight was 157. The number flashed at me and I stepped off and then back on just to make sure. I am ten pounds from goal weight. Not so long ago I almost gave up, but I have come too far not to finish this race. I want to reach that exhilarating finish line. It is time to develop a new plan, re-evaluate my progress, and develop a strategy for finishing. I have laid out the key components in "A Sprint to the Finish" contained in this book. You can apply the principles and fundamentals to your race.

Two key power phrases are helping me in these last miles to my finish line: patience and consistent obedience.

Long distance runners know the power of patience. Runners learn to pace themselves in order to have the energy and stamina needed to reach the finish line. The course, the weather, the other runners may change, but a good runner keeps the pace. In my journey, life changes happened almost every day, but finishing is still important. As a marathoner, I have needed patience as I threaded my way around other runners, patiently working my way forward. Patience helps me endure a variety of aches, pains, and inconveniences when training and running. My sprint to the finish is my last ten pounds. I believe God is going to teach me a completely new meaning for the word "patience."

The other key phrase, "consistent obedience," has resounded in my mind as I have traveled this journey. Consistent obedience is a continual process of learning and growing. We don't automatically know how to be obedient; it is something we must learn. "By faith Abraham, when called to go to a place he would later receive as his inheritance, obeyed and went, even though he did not know where he was going" (Hebrews 11:8 NIV). Abraham's faith expressed itself in obedience. He did not go in blind faith but in complete confidence in God's trustworthiness.

What is faith?

"Now faith is the assurance of things hoped for, the conviction of things not seen" (Hebrews 11:1 ESV).

Abraham heard God's voice and obeyed His words. Abraham obeyed. He focused and he obeyed. Obedience puts feet to our faith. God is calling me to finish well. I am taking a deep breath, and I am focusing on the finish line. My finish line!

I want to take you with me. Let's finish well together.

## * Personal Reflection:  Capture the Strength

I finally understand why the Lord kept whispering in my ear not to quit, not to settle for less than His very best for me, my Promised Land. Tears have cleansed my soul as God has comforted me. I find strength in His words.

"But he knows the way that I take; when he has tried me, I shall come forth as gold" (Job 23:10 ESV).

The finish line is not only in view, but it is very close. It's not over a hill or around another corner. It's right in front of me. I am aware of how much effort it is about to take to make those last few miles. Looking back is not an option.

I mentioned how I almost gave up. One day I realized the scales had not moved lately. *What is ten pounds? No one will know the difference,* I thought. Then I felt the breath of heaven press me and push me forward toward the finish line. *Joyce, don't settle for less than my best.*

The world, your family and friends may encourage you to settle where you are. "Hey, you look good. Don't get too skinny on us," they may say. But where is the place God has determined for you? He alone has a plan for you. Don't stop until you reach His goals for you, no matter how impossible it seems.

Marathons are 26.2 miles of life-changing excitement, dedicated work, deep determination, and faith. It is always a choice to train and run. Disciplined training will see you to the finish line, but not without great sacrifice and personal cost.

At the end of the marathon, runners receive a medal to remember the event. My medal is more than a physical reward. It is a mental, emotional, physical, and spiritual reward, and it has changed my life. The strength to continue and finish can only be found in the Lord. He is my strength! He will be your strength as well in your journey if you allow Him to capture your heart. Be all in!

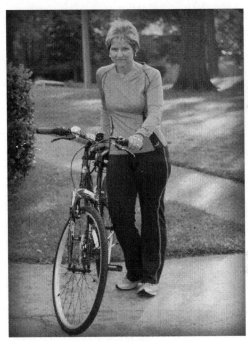

~ Joyce ~

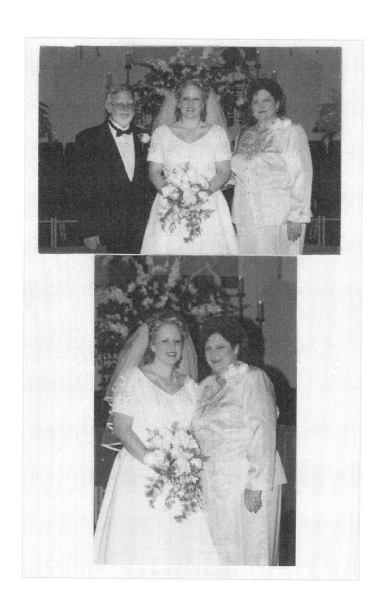

The Photos That Began Joyce's Journey

# Chapter 9
## Contagious Joy ~ Power to Continue

*As I draw near the finish, my body is tired and my muscles ache, my feet are tired and heavy. There are little patches of sodium deposits on my skin. I kind of look like an upright salt shaker. My body and clothes are wet with sweat. I feel hunger in my abdomen, and my mouth is dry and parched; I thirst for water and can feel small cracks in my lips as I wet them one more time with the tip of my tongue. Not much farther now. As I draw closer, others pass me. I push harder. I tell myself, "I can do it. I'm almost there."*

I have never been this close to making goal weight before. I'm almost there but not quite. It seems impossible. The harder I try the more determined my body is to stay at this weight. I thought my race would be easy now, but it isn't. This is where I can learn a new level of patience and consistent obedience, or should I say I can apply the patience and obedience I have learned along the way. Here is where I'll find out if the life change is for real.

I use one of those computer programs to log my food, water, and exercise for each day. At the end of the day, the computer tallies the day and computes an overview. The program predicts my weight in five weeks will be 141 pounds. Can I tell you that the computer program lies? I eat the right calories, exercise the right amount, but my weight doesn't change. I am almost to the point of throwing the computer out the window.

During my personal Bible study time one morning, I came to a familiar verse that spoke to me in a new way. The verses are about a wonderful group of Christians in the church in Ephesus. These Christians worked hard, persevered, resisted sin, and critically examined the claims of false apostles.

The church endured hardships without becoming weary. I thought how the description sounded like my weight-loss journey until I came to verse 4.

"I have this against you, that you have left your first love" (Revelation 2:1-7 NASB).

I pondered what these words meant to me and for me. Then it hit me like a ton of bricks. The FP4H program had become so much a part of my life. I learned how to measure and weigh my food, track everything I put in my mouth, stay accountable to my group, weigh in each week, complete the Bible study, memorize Scripture, and exercise daily in the FP4H program. Just as the church at Ephesus did much to benefit themselves and the community, I "did" all the correct things. But something was missing. They did good but with the wrong motive. Motive? Bingo. There it was. What was my motive?

The next morning, as I stood on my scales, I once again cried out to God. This time, however, I didn't beg Him to change the scales; instead, I renewed my commitment to Him. I said, "Lord, if these scales never move again, I will choose this day and every day henceforth to follow you."

I surrendered my heart to wait on Him to show me the finish line. When I stood on the scales, I chose to do the next right thing because I loved Jesus more than I loved food. My greatest desire from that point was to please the lover of my soul, the One who calls me precious.

I got off those scales with tears in my eyes because although I want those last ten pounds gone, I knew if I would continue to be consistently obedient that the Lord would honor my request, maybe not in my timing, but He would show me in His perfect timing the way to the finish line.

Then I had a new hope bursting in my heart and I knew that the Lord was flushing out of my spirit the last dregs of that old failure mentality. I have traded in my ashes for beauty (not a worldly beauty) and mourning has now turned to praise.

From abandoned to adored, from orphaned to adopted, from unwanted to chosen, from intense poverty to intentionally pampered. I will never have to endure the past again. I have found real freedom. He promised me a life of fulfillment and eternal rewards, even me, an adopted child. He chose me and now I choose to stay focused on the goodness of God and the countless evidences of His power, provision, protection, healing, and deliverance. There is no longer any room for doubt and unbelief.

I am filled with the hope that produces obedience and patience. I long to be so contagious with hope and joy that I will be blamed for changing people's moods and desire for a real life change, to be so consistently exuding hope and joy the atmosphere changes when I walk in the room.

I was so focused on finishing I almost missed the journey. Now my motive for finishing has changed and I am ready to develop a new kind of patience and embrace the Lord's restoration project in my life. I am all in for my lifetime.

And God began to work.

I was at church the following Sunday when one of my dear FP4H sisters said she felt like she was my Nathan. (You can read about this person in the Bible in 2 Samuel.) Nathan was a prophet. He spoke important and hard truth to King David. When David heeded Nathan's advice, great things happened. My sweet friend told me it was time to bring in reinforcements and gave me the name and number of a nutritionist.

This particular nutritionist was part of a research project involving obese patients. She did not normally see folks who had only a few pounds to lose, but with a referral from my friend, she agreed to meet with me the next week. Seeking professional help is not a sign of weakness but a sign of willingness to reach deep for the right answers. I knew I could use an unbiased opinion from sound qualified counsel.

She listened to my weight loss journey. She asked questions, evaluated my food journals, ran some tests including my weight, body measurements, body fat, BMI, as well as reviewing my previous medical records. She was appreciative of things I had learned in FP4H and encouraged me to continue living the principals of the program, but challenged me to take those principals to a new level in the coming months.

Several hours later I left her office with a revised plan of action. My first thought was rebellion; then the Lord reminded me of the declaration I had made on the scales to surrender my heart and patiently wait on Him to show me the finish line. It was as if He was saying, "I am showing you the way, now walk in obedience. Trust me on this."

Over the next few weeks, the revised plan of action began to take shape in many ways. I started by re-establishing my personal goal as well as making a recommitment to finish my journey. The scale was very important, but it should not be the only measure for me, and I acknowledged how important the whole person is. Body fat, BMI, cholesterol, triglycerides, and other numbers are all important at this stretch of the journey. I also realized how easy it is for bad habits to slip back into my life. Bad habits slip back in when we don't continually set new goals.

Next step: I had to reorganize my accountability team. The Lord brings different people into our lives in different seasons and for different reasons. I had to build a new team of people who would hold me responsible for my continuation. This was the key for me. We cannot run this race alone. If I wanted to be successful and finish, I had to give these people permission to get involved in my business in all areas --food, fitness, personal devotion time, rest, and emotional health. I don't like people up in my business, but the Lord reminded me of my commitment to patience and consistent obedience. I not only gave them permission to get in my business but I agreed to listen. Finishing was that important.

Final step: I re-evaluated my food and exercise plans under the guidance of the nutritionist's recommendations. I ate a well-balanced plan based on the FP4H guidelines, but it was time to shake my body up by moving things around. I measured and weighed my food daily. I ate most meals on my portion control plate and changed the variety and type of vegetables and fruits each day. I tried new and different foods. I even learned to like broccoli. Truly a God thing!

I focused on reducing fat and sugars in my food plan. I did not cut them out totally, because all food is permissible, but not all foods should have a prominent place in my food plan. I continued to eat at least six times a day, sometimes seven, knowing my body continually needed fuel to accomplish all it had to do.

I also re-evaluated my fitness program. I broke my exercise routine into morning and afternoon sessions. Every week I changed my rest day in my exercise routine and I tried new and different exercises, especially adding different types of cardio workouts.

Through the changes, patience with others as well as with myself proved taxing at times, but I was committed to being consistently obedient to this new level of focused attention. It is a lot easier to do the right things when we see immediate results, but by this time I was past looking for weight results. My goal was pleasing the Lord with the visible sign of my obedience, even when I saw no results.

Stepping on the scales became a weekly challenge. Would the number each week change my determination and commitment? I am not saying it did not matter, because it did and still does, but I purposed in my heart to continue to do the right things even if I did not see the right number on the scale. My place of real obedience came, not because of, but in spite of the number on the scale. I felt an extra measure of grace when the scales read 155. My new plan was working. The lower number on those scales encouraged me to press on, even though it might be painful. I was thankful for each victory loss, whether large or small. I even began to count ounces up or down. They all mattered.

In late July, I attended the FP4H Summit held each year in Houston, Texas. I love going to the Summit, traveling with friends and meeting other FP4H members who feel like extended family. The Summit is a time to fellowship, learn, grow, and encourage each other as we come together for this great two-day event. Carole Lewis, the national director of FP4H, asked me to give my testimony and an update on where I was in my journey. I was honored and stood before the crowd to tell them my story. I ended my presentation with a challenge for those present and an even bigger one for myself. I told the assembly that I intended to be at my weight goal by the end of the year and invited each person to join me at the finish line.

I wanted others to go to the finish with me; my heart wanted to see many finish their journey. I knew that many of those sweet friends had been like me, wandering around in the desert way too long or in some cases, finding the journey was too difficult. Without proper motivation and accountability, they had decided to settle east of the Jordan never quite reaching their goal. It was time to push toward the Promised Land. Many of those present decided to step out in faith and cross over the Jordan with me. Tears streamed down my face as I felt the presence of God in a new and fresh way. He breathed across my soul and a new budding hope was born.

I went home full of joy because my accountability team just got bigger and stronger. Nothing like putting a little pressure on yourself!

I am intent on walking in ever-increasing obedience to Him, so the hope I have will be an overflowing reservoir and fuel the kind of bold faith that pleases the Father. I cannot allow the enemy or my own lack of discipline or disobedience to rob me of my faith. There are many hurting people in this world, desperate for an answer to their impossible situations.

In this journey, we all run our own race and we must find our own pace. At times, we will take detours. Some of us will finish before others, but we give and receive encouragement to each other along the way. We help spur each other to the finish, needing or extending a helping hand. We need each other.

By the middle of August, the scales once again stopped moving. It was time to re-evaluate my food and fitness plan once again. I made adjustments moving food and exercise around to trigger those last few pounds to move. On September 8, 2011, I weighed in at the new session of FP4H at 154.8 pounds. I was determined and committed to walk in obedience. Teaching FP4H kept me accountable for Bible study, Scripture memorization, and weigh-in. My circle of accountability also kept me focused in the gym and on my food plan. I have never had a more loving and supportive group of friends. They helped keep me on track and focused. When I cried, they cried with me, and when I rejoiced, they rejoiced with me and for me.

My accountability partners not only encouraged, they also signed up for many of the same races and marathons. My son Daniel even trained and ran in an October half marathon with me, finishing just ahead of his mama. (I am determined to beat that boy in one of our future races together!) I challenged my accountability partners with several events I named as "a real challenge to change." I said the challenge would be fun. They joined in for the opportunity to encourage me (I told them they were all just "medal" happy, because at every event we get a medal if we participate, not just the top winners).

During that October half marathon, I met Patrick House, one of the winners from *The Biggest Loser* show. He walked/ran the half marathon, too. After we crossed the finish line I teased, "Patrick, I finished before you." We laughed together and had a wonderful conversation about our common bond of weight loss and our deep desire not to return to our old ways. We had our photo made together. He is a nice person.

After the race, I attended a victory party, which was actually a surprise birthday party for me. I was going to turn 51 on October 21. My friends surprised me, but thankfully, they did not give me a cake, just great food, fellowship, and some fabulous gifts.

The only thing that could have made the party better would have been me reaching my goal weight. By the middle of October, I stepped on the scales and saw 153 flash at me. I stepped off and back on just to make sure. Not much farther now.

I was about to enter the toughest two months of the year: November and December. My husband, our two very best friends, and I signed up for a half marathon in January. At first I thought I must be out of my mind. I hate cold weather, and the weather for this half marathon had been twenty degrees the previous year. I thought perhaps I needed to get my head examined instead of my body, but my best friend reminded me training for this marathon would take place during the months when food choices could be difficult.

With another half marathon and holiday months ahead, it was time to re-evaluate my food and exercise plans, establish a training schedule for the half marathon, and set the pace for the finish. I was totally surrendered at that point to the work Christ was doing in my life. By November 10, I weighed 150.6 pounds. Only fifty-one days before the end of the year and 3.4 pounds from goal. Could I finish? Was it possible?

I realized more than ever that freedom cost something. In order to celebrate success and finally finish I had to be willing to pay the price that success required. Truth is I couldn't do it. I did not have it in me, but Christ did.

"But we have this treasure in earthen vessels, so that the surpassing greatness of the power will be of God and not from ourselves" (2 Corinthians 4:7 NASB).

My human weakness was going to provide the occasion for the triumph of divine power. When I finally stepped over the finish line, there would be no doubt in my mind "Who" accomplished this victory in my life. I chose freedom one more time; whatever the cost, I was in to the finish.

Then the enemy's old familiar voice whispered, "What if the scales never move down another pound, Joyce? What if you don't make goal by the end of the year?"

Then God asked, "Will you go back? Will you stop being obedient?"

Grace is unmerited favor. Like all humans, I was born into spiritual poverty without a hint of hope on my own ability, but God saw me and His heart was moved to travel from heaven to earth and from a throne to a cross to extend His hand of grace. He saw me as precious, and the reply from my heart, full of His unmerited favor, was love. The last chain of bondage finally broke and freedom was complete. I am still in, Lord; I am still in, Lord, all the way.

## * Personal Reflection: Celebrate the Victory

Patience and consistent obedience became my best friends during this part of my journey. I had to learn to be patient in the journey not only with myself and others, but also with the Lord, learning to surrender daily to the work that He was perfecting in me and allowing Him to lead and me follow.

Seeking help and advice from professionals is also an important aspect in the journey. We have to also put into action what needs to be done. It is a decision followed by a process.

Be willing to finish! Finishing is just the beginning of the journey. Through the process of finishing, we learn how to continue to choose well daily. In order to celebrate success and finally finish I had to be willing to pay the price that success required, and so do you.

My life change process had to be a priority for me regardless of what it cost. Change is going to cost something! Be willing to pay the price. You are worth it.

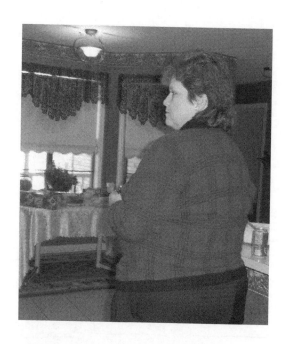

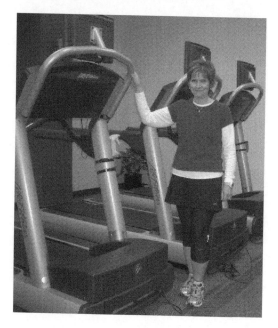

Joyce – Before and After

# Chapter 10
## The Finish Line – Reach Your Goal

*At mile ten, I felt a pain. It was not too bad, just a slight stitch in the left hip and side, but now, with just 3.4 miles to go, the pain is almost unbearable, a sharp, shooting pain in the worst way. I've tried everything—altered my breathing, slowed my pace, tried pushing off from my right leg, but nothing seems to help. The only thing good about this pain is how it makes all my other aches and pains appear more bearable. I feel a constant sting of sweat in my eyes. The skin on my feet is raw; I know I am beyond the help of Vaseline, skin sake, or body glide. My blisters have formed, broken, and are now bleeding and painful with every step.*

*The muscles that ached and hurt miles back are now numb. There is no feeling left. I wondered if runners ever "hit the wall" twice in one race. No, perhaps I am hallucinating. Months of training never prepared me for this. Then I look up and see my friends and family, my encouragers. I am almost there.*

*Suddenly a gust of crosswind causes me to stumble. Then as if invisible hands straighten out my flimsy legs, I am able to regain my form. One more corner and I'll reach the last water station. Just two more miles to go. I reach for a cup from the volunteer. She smiles an angelic smile and says, "You are almost there. You can do it. Keep going. Finish strong." I slow my pace enough to drink the refreshing water while I reach for another one. I pour it over my head, grab a final cup, and add its contents to the one streaming down my head, back, and arms.*

*I step back in the flow of runners and press on. Crushed and discarded paper cups crumple under each painful step. Leg cramps begin in my lower leg and move upward toward my thigh. I pull out my final pack of mustard. I don't know how or why it works, but mustard gives relief from leg cramps.*

*With cracked and parched lips, I tear the packet open. "Lord, help the pain subside." I can't let anything stop me. I have to finish.*

*Cheering crowds line the streets. Words of encouragement fade as the faces blur; just one more mile to go. With one agonizing step after another, gasping for breath with a mouth of cotton and dried mustard, running on legs of lead with pain in every muscle and joint, I press on. The cramps begin to ease. Thank you, Jesus. When I think I cannot take another step, the next song comes on my iPod, a song I need to hear one more time.*

*The lyrics remind me how Christ has been with me through every step of the race. I sing and cry at the same time and remember Psalm 139.*

*O LORD, You have searched me and known me.*

*You know when I sit down and when I rise up;*

*You understand my thought from afar.*

*You scrutinize my path and my lying down,*

*And are intimately acquainted with all my ways.*

*Even before there is a word on my tongue,*

*Behold, O LORD, You know it all.*

*You have enclosed me behind and before,*

*And laid Your hand upon me.*

*Such knowledge is too wonderful for me;*

*It is too high, I cannot attain to it. (Psalm 139:1-6 NASB).*

*In a crowd of runners and spectators, I have a quiet, still moment with my Savior. I see His face and know He loves me. I am precious to Him.*

*Then I see it. Penned in large letters, hanging above the street, the word I have longed to see – FINISH LINE.*

*Mustering every ounce of strength, I press through the other runners. I hear the announcer call out the names of finishers.*

*"I can finish strong."* I block out the aches and pains, push harder, and then hear people cheering. I smile. Only a little farther. I move steadily through the last strides of the torturous journey, determined to sprint to the end. I stand tall, shoulders back, head high . . . and then, I hear my name. With arms raised high in triumph, I cross the finish line!

And the scales announced the good news. My goal weight: 147 pounds! I thanked God for the ability to finish. For through Him all things are truly possible.

I finally made goal weight of 147 pounds. I tell friends you have to hold a weight loss for three consecutive days before you can count it as real. Three days later, I had maintained my goal weight. More important than the number on the scale (yes, I said that) was my BMI, which dropped to 24.9 (into the normal range) and my body fat was finally at a 29.2 (also in the normal range). Both BMI and body fat had dropped considerably over the last month of my journey. I had someone from my gym track all measurements and numbers for me, not trusting myself to be completely accurate in this critical place of my journey.

I am smaller now than when I was twelve years old. Humbling is all I can say, very humbling.

In January my husband, two very close friends, and I ran the Blues half marathon. I had prayed for warm weather that day and guess what. I got it. The weather was cool but nice and unseasonably warm for a Mississippi January. God is so good. As usual, my husband and friends finished before me, but you know what is so sweet? They all came back for me.

They found me about two miles out with a painful limp, leg cramps, out of mustard, and tears streaming down my face. They came alongside me and ran with me to the finish line. I made it.[2]

---

[2] Thank you, Donna, for being my pacer those last two miles. I love you, my friend. I could not have done it without you.

## * Personal Reflections:  Finish the Race

There were some critical factors in my last ten pounds to goal weight. I have included a tip sheet in the appendix called *Sprint to the Finish*. I hope these pointers will help you find the keys to unlock the door for your finish line. The last ten pounds were by far the hardest to lose.

Lately, I have been pondering the truth of Isaiah 40:31: "But they that wait upon the Lord shall renew their strength; they shall mount up with wings as eagles; they shall run, and not be weary; and they shall walk, and not faint" (KJV).

I have finally found freedom. I am still in, Lord, all the way. Now it's time to build a heritage of lasting life change and help others find that same freedom.

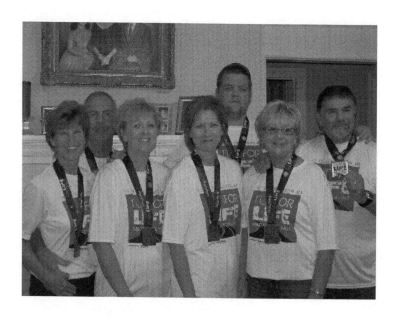

Run for Life Half Marathon ~ Helping others find freedom

# Chapter 11
## Build a Heritage of Life Change ~ Help Others Find Freedom

Every runner knows the thrill of seeing the finish line. Whether the run is a 5K, a 10K, a 12K, a half marathon or even a 26.2-mile full marathon, the sight of the finish line motivates us to push, to sprint, and to finish strong. No matter how exhausted we feel, something happens when we see the finish line. In several marathons, the race officials take my friend Donna directly to the medical tent after crossing the finish line. She expends her last ounce of energy both physically and emotionally because she sprints to the finish line with hands raised in victory and triumph.

At the finish line, one of the first things you notice is your time. In most races they post it just over your head. Time is not that important to me. I am just thankful I did not give up or quit. One hundred ninety-two pounds has been a long journey. How far I have come the last few years! Not an easy journey, but a completed journey. My body is in excellent shape and I continue to push it to endure more.

My spirit is soaring. My walk with the Lord is closer than it has ever been. I have entered the Promised Land and am learning to live here. I have learned to walk daily every step of the way—not every mile but every step with Him. My life is truly a journey, a marathon not a sprint. I allow Him to lead, and I find He is able to use all the things in my life, even the detours and valleys, for joy. I can, by His power and strength, accomplish the impossible.

The children of Israel built a memorial with the stones taken from the bed of the Jordan River as a constant reminder of the day the Israelites crossed over on dry ground (See Joshua 4.) As they walked in faith and obedience, the nation was forever changed. The memorial was a constant reminder of God's miracle.

Along my journey, I have picked up memorial stones, too. I have recovered from the emotional and physical scars of compulsive eating and overeating. Now I want to position my memorial in a place and in such a way I will be constantly reminded of my life change process. Going back will never be an option.

My memorial stones are a reminder to me and to others that a life of freedom is truly possible and attainable. I not only want to build a memorial, but I want to build a heritage of life change. I want to help my own family, as well as many others, find this same place of freedom in their lives. So the question is, how does that happen? Let's take a look at my memorial stones.

## The Stone of Truth

The Stone of Truth is the foundational stone. Everything about the life-change process begins with truth. I have gained great understanding about God's plans for me over the last few years. The Bible says, "Who is the Man who fears the Lord? He (the Lord) will instruct him (me) in the way he should choose. His (my) soul will abide in prosperity, and his (my) descendants will inherit the land. The secret of the Lord is for those who fear (hold Him in high regard) Him (Christ) (Psalm 25: 12-14 NASB) (parentheses mine).

Fearing God means recognizing God is holy, almighty, righteous, pure, all-knowing, all-powerful, and all wise. When I regard God correctly, I gain a clearer picture of myself. I was and I am still weak, sinful, frail, and desperately needy. I am unable to make the right decisions or choices daily on my own.

Humble respect is due the Lord—to Him and for Him. Reverence, or to use the biblical word "fear," allows me to acknowledge I am totally dependent on Him. Life change is not possible without His strength and power. I allowed food a powerful position in my life, but the power and strength of the Lord broke the chains of bondage.

## The Stone of Surrender

The second stone in my memorial is the Stone of Surrender. I chose to surrender my mind and body to the truth that has set me free. I don't think the same way about food or exercise anymore. I don't see things the same way either. Now, I want you to hear me on this. I love to eat and I enjoy eating. I don't eat food I don't like (unhealthy or healthy). Food has a place in my life, but it no longer has a place of power. I choose the healthiest thing I can possibly eat because I now have a deep desire to honor my body instead of heap abuse on it from poor food choices. I believe when I make choices, I choose life or death. Choosing wisely is life and choosing poorly is death.

Can I be real here? This is a process. I did not get to this place overnight. I am the girl that enjoyed eating a dozen Krispy Crème donuts with the cream filling. One donut made me mad; it never was enough. But I refuse to apologize for the fact that I no longer desire to have any Krispy Crème donuts. Not one. Not because I can't, because I can. I have no desire for one. That does not make me weird. It is a God thing, a God thing I am thankful has happened.

Of course, at times, I do choose poorly. I am human. I also have certain foods I have always enjoyed, like ice cream. I still enjoy ice cream and have it on a regular basis. I figured out a way to add ice cream into my plan. This way I can make wise choices and still enjoy foods I love. There is no guilt or condemnation for enjoying ice cream because it is part of the plan.

Exercise is also another area requiring surrender. I often try to talk myself out of going to the gym. If it were not for my accountability group, I would falter in this area. Some days I love going and some days I don't. I am thankful for the days I love to go, and on the days I don't, I am thankful for a team who will not allow me to quit. I surrender because I know it is the right thing to do, not because I feel like it. I remind myself how fickle feelings are and I don't allow feelings to lead me down the wrong path or into a detour. Every choice to surrender makes the next choice easier. Each surrender helps me enjoy the right choices. The key is surrender. Choose every day to do the next right thing. Guarding my mind is a vital part of the life change process. And it begins with daily surrender.

## The Stone of Accountability

The Stone of Accountability is, and will continue to be, an absolute must for me. My memorial cannot stand without this critical component. I want to keep my mind focused on freedom instead of failure. According to an old saying, "amateurs train until they get it right, while professionals train until they can't get it wrong."

The question is, do I want to be an amateur who does just enough to get by, or do I want to be a professional who trains so well I will do the right thing without hesitation? There are three keys to reach this level of success: knowledge, practice, and coaching.

Knowledge is gained by studying. Learn the right foods and food combinations. Understand which exercises build muscle and reduce fat. Understand the physical and emotional steps to success. We can also gain knowledge by sharing life with others. Hang out with someone who models good, healthy, positive life change and hang out with him or her on a regular basis.

The next step after gaining knowledge is to practice what we know, because to know and not do is sin (See James 4:17). The key is keeping on. Keep doing it. Again and again. The first time I went to a Body Pump class, I felt stupid. *This is not for me. This is really a waste of my time.* The next morning I could not get out of bed. Every body part hurt and was sore. I realized the benefit of the class. Maybe, just maybe, I was out of shape. I went back and kept going back. I still go and now I love Body Pump. I don't like getting up at 4:30 a.m. to participate, but I love the way I feel after the class and I am done.

The final key to success is coaching. We need someone to help us along in the process of life change, someone who is willing to walk alongside to encourage, direct, and correct. It takes a huge act of courage to be vulnerable enough to allow someone into our lives. Someone that will see the good, the bad, and the ugly. But when we make ourselves vulnerable, we grow, and we impact those around us. We have to learn to be willing to reach out and ask for help and advice. First Place 4 Health has been my coach. We are in this together, and I don't want to go back. I don't want you to go back either. Not ever. Practicing the principals of the life change process together will ensure our continued success.

## The Stone of Obedience

The final memorial stone I want to lay down is the Stone of Obedience. It is at the top of my memorial for a reason. None of the other stones is as useful or powerful without the Stone of Obedience. I continue to practice the components of life change daily and the act of obedience ensures that I do … on the days I feel like it and on the days I don't feel like it.

My memorial is now in place. Three large stones. Truth. Surrender. Obedience.

So what now? I've identified two elements to long-term life change success.

My first new goal is to live life fully. I want to live the good life, but I still have to have a plan. On this side of the finish line, I look back, evaluate what worked, and continue to do those things. The valuable lessons I've learned helped me cross the finish line and will give me the tools and strength to live here and never go back.

If I put down deep roots in the Promised Land, I can weather the storms without giving up my new way of life. I never want to default back to the old failure mentality or to my poor habits that caused me to get off track and lose my pace. I want to be able to run with endurance.

Sometimes it's not the storms but the winds of change or discontentment that erode our good intentions and healthy lifestyle. If we are mindful of this, we can prevent it from happening. Not too long ago, I spent an afternoon walking on the beach, when a strong wind picked up, blowing sand up, hitting my feet and legs until it became painful. I finally gave up on the walk and returned indoors. The next morning when I returned to the beach, the sand and dunes from the day before had shifted.

Think about how each small grain of sand moved almost imperceptibly but the landscape changed dramatically. The little things in my life and in your life affect the big picture. You work late. You feel tired. You have a fight with your spouse. You develop a cold. Your regular routine is disrupted. Your kids or grandkids have a ball game. You develop an injury. You don't like the temperature in the church, the pastor doesn't seem to be preaching as well as he once did, or he keeps preaching the same thing over and over. You take a vacation or work out of town a few weeks or a weekend. A dear friend goes into the hospital. There is a death in the family. It is raining. It is just too cold. The list goes on and on.

Little grains of stress, discontent, dissatisfaction, a poor choice here, and a bad choice there and then one morning we wake up late and decide quiet time with the Lord is too much effort and eating right and making healthy choices is not as easy as it used to be, or exercise has become like work again. Little grains of sand change the whole picture. Our life change deteriorates into the same old habits. Little disturbances or interruptions destroy our great accomplishments. We need a plan to deal with the little changes. Decide now how you will identify and address stress if you will be successful at real life change.

My second new goal is to help others. I am compelled to help others find the way to real life change. How will what I've learned help someone else who is beginning the race?

Before my last half marathon, I said to my husband, "I'm not sure why I keep signing up for these crazy races. I love the challenge of training but hate the race itself." But I encouraged him and my other runner friends to do their best, knowing they would run faster than I would.

During the race, I was running alone. I don't really like running on my own, because I enjoy talking to someone as I run. The damp asphalt road stretched out endlessly in front of me. I struggled up every incline, and fought the desire to quit almost every step of the race. I didn't realize we had so many stinking hills in downtown Jackson. I had trained for this, I had eaten correctly, and I had stayed on my plan through the holidays. I thought I should enjoy this race. I should be able to breeze through this, but I am a whiner. Can you tell? It appeared that I had done all the right things, but why wasn't this easier?

Do you see the problem? Mindset. I had the wrong expectation. Races are hard, and sometimes the shortest ones can be the hardest. They are supposed to be a measure of endurance and hard work. Half marathons and marathons are uniquely grueling because of the emotional impact as well as the physical impact on the body. Where did I ever get the idea that race day was going to be easy? I had a mental picture of a breezy show of athletic prowess and pride floating over the finish line as everyone cheered.

As I plowed up the hill at Lefluer's Bluff in the middle of the race, I wondered how often in my life I had the same idea about God's blessings. I expect His blessings to be largely about my personal comfort and expect blessings to come because I walk in obedience.

Running on empty and feeling very tired, I hung my head. I wanted to quit. When I looked up, there they were. My husband. My best friends. Running alongside me, encouraging me, and telling me I was doing great. Tears came to my eyes and I knew I could finish.

God had been with me through it all, but He sent reinforcements. Through FP4H and my friends and family, God has run alongside me. My goal now is to cheer and urge and encourage others to make life changes that matter.

Crossing the finish line was just the beginning, not the end. Reaching my weight-loss goal is a precarious place for me. I have never been here before and I have to learn how to live here. I have been in weight-loss "mind mode" for years now. What now?

After a couple of weeks in maintenance land, I e-mailed my nutritionist to give her a run--down of my numbers. I asked, "Do you think I need to lose a few more pounds?" It did not take her long to respond. "No."

Her answer was plain, simple, and I had no problem understanding her. I needed to learn how to live in a place of maintenance. I have a feeling there will be other interesting challenges, races and even a few detours in this journey; in this life-change process. I am excited about what might be next.

Truth, surrender, accountability, and obedience are the stones of my memorial to life change. I am committed to guarding my heart and mind against wrong expectations and discontentment by training myself and allowing others to hold me accountable in the process. I am committed to continually seeking knowledge, wisdom, and guidance from God and others. Practicing life change and seeking out the right coaching as well as being a coach to others in this journey until I am no longer an amateur but a professional.

I want to make a difference in the lives of others so that the heritage I pass on will be one of hope, help, and healing. I plan to continue setting goals for myself and encouraging others to do the same. By God's strength we will not only walk but run in freedom.

## * Personal Reflections: Encourage Others

What a race! Starting line of 339 pounds and finish line at 147 pounds. I still look in the mirror expecting to see that other 192 pounds. I pray that as I continue to walk in obedience the Lord will remove all traces of that image from my mind.

I keep pictures of the old me as part of my memorial, of where I have come from and where I am determined never to return. We all need reminders of the past but that is what they need to be just reminders. Don't focus so much on where you have come from that you miss where you are going. Focus on your finish line.

In this book, I have included a personal evaluation form designed to help you be honest and get on track as well as a 21-Day Jump Start Plan. I have also included some helpful resources; a study guide has now been added for those wanting to use this as a small group study and websites that will give you guidance for success. Also included is a copy of the Positive Affirmations I said daily and A Sprint to the Finish plan that will help you lose those last few stubborn pounds. You will also find a list of healthy tips on food and exercise. These tips really worked for me; I hope you'll find them helpful. These tools and resources are for you. You "Can" lose the weight and experience life change. You Can! By the power of Christ.

"I have fought the good fight, I have finished the race, I have kept the faith" (2 Timothy 4:7 NASB)

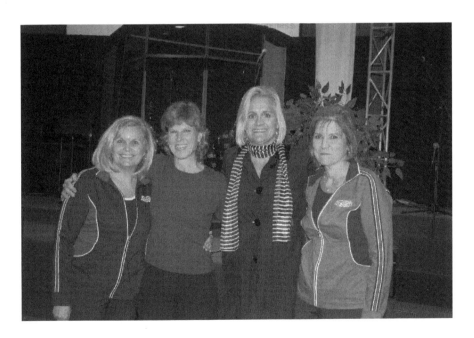

Hope for You Event ~ Joyce with Vicki Heath (far left), Donna, Becky Turner (far right next to Joyce)

# Personal Evaluation

## Where Are You?

For real life change to happen and for us to receive help in these areas of weakness in our life we must be willing to tell ourselves the truth and reach out for help. We cannot change what we are unwilling to admit.

Please truthfully answer the following questions concerning where you are in the journey. Whether you have a great deal of weight to lose or just those last few stubborn pounds, or maybe you struggle with some other type of bondage or addiction, taking a personal evaluation will help you track where you are and what needs to change for you to get to your finish line.

How long have I been overweight or in bondage? _20+ years_

    If your addiction is not to food please list it here _____

Please name your addiction. Remember we cannot change what we do not acknowledge.

What weight-loss or addiction programs have I started before?
_Weight Watchers, First Place, weight loss doctor, many weight-loss books_

How many times?
_Too many to count_

Do I have someone weigh me each week?
_Yes._

Do I track my food <u>daily</u> and <u>accurately</u>?
_Just starting to do this_

Have I identified my "trigger" foods in my eating patterns (do I have a particular food that causes me to fall off my plan from time to time/ a food I have a specific weakness for?)

_Sweets_

Do I have a personal accountability partner that I can talk with about anything? Someone who is willing to help me stay on track?

_No - 4·28·16 asked Brooke_

Do I have a regular (daily) exercise program? _Not yet - working on getting one - setting goals_

What do you feel is your weakest area of the "life change" process that holds you back from either overcoming this addiction, losing weight or losing those last few pounds?

_Falling back into old habits of handling stress; feeling like it's "impossible"_

Do I have a regular support group, Bible study group, or accountability program that I go to weekly for support and help for this area in my life? _Yes - thank you, Lord for this First Place group!_

Do you read and study your Bible or have a quite time on a daily basis?

_Yes_

Do you feel stuck? If so, do you know why?

_Yes - because I have tried and failed so many times (on my own)_

Do I really desire real and lasting change in my life?

_Yes !_

Am I willing to "do" what it will take to finally find freedom?

_Yes_

Now prayerfully consider your answers. Then meet with a friend, pastor, or an accountability partner. Allow someone to help you.

# Fast Facts for Personal Evaluation Assessment

We cannot begin in the right place if we do not acknowledge where we are. A personal evaluation of where we have been and where we are is a **must** if we really want to meet our personal goals.

Seek professional help, a trusted advisor, counselor, fitness expert, life coach, or nutritionist. (I hired a nutritionist to give me some expert advice and help me re-evaluate my plan. I also have a personal trainer at my local gym.)

## Fact 1: Re-evaluate

After you take a personal evaluation, ask someone you trust to go over the evaluation with you. Make assessments in all the areas (mental, emotional, spiritual, and physical.)

## Fact 2: Re-establish

Make sure your personal goal is doable and reachable. Bad habits have a way of pushing back into our life when we stop setting goals for ourselves. Focus on the goals. Get off the "diet" merry-go-round and focus on a healthy new lifestyle.

## Fact 3: Re-organize

Share your information with a trusted accountability partner. (Build a team of accountability around yourself.) The Lord brings different people into our lives in different seasons and for different reasons. An accountability partner is a must. If you don't have one, begin praying for one now. We cannot do this alone. Give your accountability partners permission to get in your business, in all areas, if you want to be successful and finish strong.

**Fact 4: <u>Re-vamp</u>**

Occasionally give your program a facelift. Sometimes it is just a matter of moving things around in the day, eating different foods, or exercising at different times. We may need to add a support group to our plan. The key is to do something different.

**Fact 5: <u>Re-commit</u>**

Plan to complete your journey. Make some changes and keep making changes until you figure out what is going to work for you. Do whatever it takes to finish, and take someone with you to the finish line.

**Truth:**

We must willingly choose freedom. Freedom costs. In order to celebrate success we have to be willing to pay the price success requires. We can't do it, but He can.

**Truth:**

"But we have this treasure in earthen vessels, so that the surpassing greatness of the power will be of God and not from ourselves" (2 Corinthians 4:7 NASB). Our human weakness provides the occasion for the triumph of divine power. Allow Christ to shine through you.

**Truth:**

True joy comes from a consistent relationship with Jesus Christ. When our lives are intertwined with His, our joy will be evident in the good times and the tough times regardless of our circumstances because of our daily walk with Christ. Remember, He is the one who gives us the strength.

# Helpful Resources and Websites for Success

I am a firm believer in using all the help available. Fortunately, we have the Internet as a wonderful resource for success. The following resources and websites were useful "tools" for my life change. With your hard work and diligence and these helpful tools, you can and will be successful.

**Portion Control Plate**: I love this plate! Much of my success came because I used this tool. The plate is divided into sections to help you control your portions. Studies show people who use the portion control plate method not only lose weight but also learn to keep it off because they discover the value of portion control. The plate is portable enough to be used at work, home, or even in a restaurant. It is versatile enough for children and adults.

The portion control plate comes with directions (my plate method plan) I call it and a "sample day" of meals just to help get you started. At this time my portion control plate can only be ordered from my website so visit me at **www.joyceainsworth.com** or you can also contact me at **glenna@netdoor.com** for pricing and special discounts for bulk or group orders.

**Food Scale**: Weighing food helps with portion control. Knowing the exact portion will help you get on track and stay on track. Order the food scale at **glenna@netdoor.com** or **www.joyceainsworth.com**.

**Strength and Flexibility Bands**: I love the variety of exercises I can do with these wonderful bands. They are great for travel, work, gym, or home fitness plans. Fitness bands are available in many variations. The ones I recommend can be used to work every major muscle group in the body. Regardless of sport or fitness level, strength and flexibility bands are a great addition that you need to fit into your workout regimen. These can be ordered from all sorts of websites.

## Helpful Websites for Success

+ For all types of information and resources: **www.firstplace4health.com**
+ Healthy weight calculator: **www.cdc.gov/healthyweight/assessing/bmi**
+ Center for Disease Control: **www.CDC.gov**
+ 2010 Dietary Guidelines: **www.DietaryGuidelines.gov**
+ Brochure with tips on how to build your plate: **www.choosemyplate.gov/food-groups/downloads/MyPlate/DG2010Brochure.pdf**
+ A government website where you will find information and tools to help you and those you care about stay healthy: **www.healthfinder.gov**
+ Physical Activity Guidelines for Americans: **http://www.health.gov/paguidelines**
+ How to read the nutrition facts panel: **http://www.fda.gov/Food/ResourcesForYou/Consumers/NFLPM/ucm274593.htm**
+ National Heart, Lung, and Blood Institute Obesity Education Initiative: **http://www.nhlbi.nih.gov/about/oei/index.htm** (Portion Distortion quiz, etc.)
+ First lady's childhood obesity initiative: **www.letsmove.gov**
+ USDA site to help with goals and improve the nutrition and well-being of Americans, June 2011 ("my plate" replaced "my pyramid"): **www.choosemyplate.gov**
+ Healthy eating on a budget: **www.choosemyplate.gov/healthy-eating-on-budget.html**

- FP4H online tracker: **www.firstplace4health.com**
- Other trackers: **www.mypyramidtracker.gov, www.myfitnesspal.com, www.livestrong.com, www.calorieking.com**
- Kids' food tracking worksheet: **http://teamnutrition.usda.gov/resources/mpk_worksheet.pdf**
- Healthy tips for families: **http://teamnutrition.usda.gov/Resources/mpk_tips.pdf**
- Tips to cut back on kids' sweets treats: **http://www.choosemyplate.gov/food-groups/downloads/TenTips/DGTipsheet13CutBackOnSweetTreats.pdf**
- Tips for making healthy foods more fun for children: **http://www.choosemyplate.gov/food-groups/downloads/TenTips/DGTipsheet11KidFriendlyVeggiesAndFruits.pdf**
- To learn the amount of each food group you need daily by age, weight, and gender: **http://www.choosemyplate.gov/myplate/index.aspx**
- Tips to be a healthy role model for children: **http://www.choosemyplate.gov/food-groups/downloads/TenTips/DGTipsheet12BeAHealthyRoleModel.pdf**
- National Christian weight loss program: **www.firstplace4health.com**
- Info on tools to help you stay healthy: **http://www.healthfinder.gov**
- Products that enhance exercise: **www.jeffgalloway.com** or **www.phidippides.com**

- ✦ The world's largest organization of food and nutrition professionals, formerly the American Dietetic Association: **www.eatright.org**
- ✦ Consumer reporting for health products: **www.consumerlab.com**
- ✦ Science and health info: **www.tcolincampbell.org/courses-resources/home**[ii]
- ✦ A great website that helps you find healthier food options than the ones you are using and also helps you create a personal grocery list: **www.shopwell.com**
- ✦ A great on-line bakery for the health and allergy conscious where you can find and buy healthy options foods: **Sami'sbakery.com**
- ✦ A great app that can be downloaded to help you grade foods in the grocery store and also gives you nutrition facts about that product.

Visit the app store on your phone and look for **fooducate** There are other health and fitness apps that can now be bought and downloaded to your phone that will be a great resource for your new lifestyle that have great health benefits. Check out the options available to you in the app store on your device.

# 21-Day Jump Start Plan

Most of us struggle in the beginning. Life change is hard, but getting started is harder than running the race. So, here is a 21-day jump-start to help you get on track and in the race. Please remember this is not a perfect science and the real key is to make this a personal plan adapted to you and your specific needs. Don't go on a "diet." Start thinking about a new lifestyle. Thinking about learning and choosing to be healthy will get you headed in a new direction.

## The Seven Steps to Preparation:

The seven steps to preparation is the process of cleaning the home, body, and mind of "junk." These are critical steps you need for the life change process to begin. This is simply your jump-start; your starting point. Here you will establish clear priorities to guide your steps and actions. Preparation will allow you to complete your journey. So it is time. Start now.

**Step 1:** Be willing to have someone weigh you each week. This is a must and not an option. You have many choices on who can do this; a trainer at the gym, your doctor's office, a fitness group or your accountability team. Weigh-in should be about the same time and day each week. One friend weighs on her scale on Tuesday morning and sends me a picture of the scale. Yes it is that important. Track your weight loss progress.

**Step 2:** Clean out your kitchen, including your refrigerator and pantry. If you don't buy it and bring it into the house, you will not be tempted to eat it. Just say "no" to all junk food. Make your home a haven of healthy food choices. Choose well these first few weeks and avoid the food items that are the most tempting by not allowing them in your home. Clean your car and desk at work as well. Doing this will make choosing well an easier choice in the coming weeks.

**Step 3**: Portion control plate: If you don't have one, buy one. Eating from a portion control plate will be one of your greatest tools the first few weeks. Until you really learn and understand a solid food plan, the portion plate will make a difference. You can order my plate from my website **www.joyceainsworth.com**

**Step 4**: Accountability partner: You need someone who can and will help you in your journey. We all need a buddy; so find a buddy. Find someone who is willing to hold you accountable in the areas of eating and exercise. This person needs to be someone who loves you enough to tell you the truth, not be your partner in crime. Someone who is also committed to making a life change will make a great accountability partner.

**Step 5**: Join a group: My preference is FP4H, but everyone needs to be involved in a support group of one type or another. You need to be connected. Individuals who are part of a group have a higher success rate. People who say, "I can do this on my own," usually fail. We were created for community. We are wired for relationship. So find or start a group of some kind. Health and fitness groups are becoming very popular now days.

**Step 6**: Learn to track your food. This process is an absolute must. Individuals who track their food intake are more successful at weight loss. There are lots of great websites and apps to help you. Write it down in a book, on your phone, I Pad, laptop, or home PC. Just do it.

**Step 7**: Commit to a fitness program. The road to poor health is paved with good intentions. Exercise has to have a place of high priority in your schedule and your new lifestyle. Physical fitness requires the discipline to exercise regularly. So start somewhere. Start with 30 minutes a day. Adding in the fitness component is critical to your success. Don't wait. Start now.

# Food for a Lifetime
## 21-Day Jump Start

Healthy eating begins with good food choices daily. In twenty-one days, the good choices will become good habits. Getting started is not a perfect science and the real key is to make this a personal plan adapted to you and your specific needs. Don't go on a diet. Instead, start making some new positive food choices. Food, just like exercise, should be approached with the principals of balance, variety, and moderation. Here are a few healthy tips to help you get started.

### Tip 1:

Establish a well-balanced food plan and know your calorie range. Your plan should include all of the following in proper balance. Focus on eating more fruits and vegetables. Your goal is to learn how to make healthy, low-fat food choices. Be willing to cut out the junk. Avoid high fat foods (especially fried and sugary foods). These foods have no real value to the body, so if you are serious about making a change, avoid these foods, especially at the beginning.

    A. Carbohydrates: The largest percentage of your total calories should come from carbohydrates. These foods break down into glucose, the main fuel your brain and muscles use. In addition to supplying energy, carbohydrates such as whole grains, beans, fruits, and vegetables also supply vitamins, minerals, and dietary fiber.

    B. Proteins: Most of us actually get way too much protein every day. We have a hard time choosing quality protein-rich foods. By choosing meat low in saturated fat and cholesterol, as well as incorporating vegetarian sources of protein into your food intake, you can provide your body with the nutrients it needs for maintenance and repair, but save yourself added fat, cholesterol, and calories. Good healthy protein choices can be found in the following: lean meats, poultry, fish, eggs, low or non-fat dairy products, and vegetable proteins like beans, tofu, or legumes.

C. Fats: Although fat is an essential nutrient, much of the fat we consume is unnecessary for good nutrition. Focus on what I call healthy fats and good oils. Monounsaturated fat is found in olive oil, peanut oil, canola oil, avocados, poultry, nuts, and seeds. Some examples of polyunsaturated fat are vegetable oils (such as safflower, corn, sunflower, soy, and cottonseed oils), nut oils (such as peanut oil), poultry, nuts, and seeds. Omega-3 fatty acids include choices such as cold-water fish (salmon, mackerel, and herring), ground flaxseed, flaxseed oil, and walnuts.
The fats we need to watch for and avoid are saturated fats, trans fats, and hydrogenated vegetable oils.

D. Water: Water is the most vital nutrient your body needs. Every cell depends on water to function. Water is your body's principal chemical component and makes up about 60 percent of your body weight. Water is essential for the digestion and absorption of food. It also flushes toxins out of vital organs, carries nutrients to your cells, and is vital in the elimination of digestive waste.

## Tip 2:
Don't skip meals and always eat breakfast. Skipping meals isn't healthy and is not a sensible way to lose weight. Focus on eating three smaller meals a day and two or three healthy snacks (use your portion control plate). Remember moderation and variety.

**Sample of an eating plan for one day:**

Breakfast: One 6-ounce yogurt/small fruit/coffee, hot tea, or warm lemon water (women's calorie target should be 200 to 300 calories. Men should be in the 300 to 400 calorie range).

Mid-Morning Snack: Snacks should be less than 200 calories (even for men). Some suggestions include protein bars, peanut butter and crackers, Kashi granola bars, or Kellogg's Fiber One bar.

Caution: The main thing to remember on snacks is to avoid high sugar or high fat items. Read the labels even on protein bars and granola bars. Some brands are packed with sugar and fat. Find a good quality food to have as a snack, but try to make sure it contains some solid protein and good carbohydrates.

Lunch: Plate Method: Review plate method handout included in each portion-controlled plate package. Choose foods from all food groups and choose balance.

Mid-afternoon Snack: Should be 100 calories or less. A great snack for mid-afternoon is a 1-ounce cheese stick, cocoa-dusted almonds in the 100-calorie pack, or a 6-ounce carb-master yogurt. Always look for quality foods for snacks.

Dinner: Plate Method: Review plate method handout. Choose foods from all food groups and choose balance.

After-dinner or Bedtime Snack: Eat a very light snack (cup of baby carrots, milk, or fruit held over from dinner). If this is a snack you feel you need, target making it less than 100 calories, preferably 80 calories or less. (A great little snack would be a Healthy Choice fudge sickle at about 80 calories). Yes you can still have ice cream!

## Tip 3:

Use the step-down program to replace unhealthy habits with healthy living. Removing unhealthy habits without replacing them with healthy habits causes us to be negative and have a depravation mentality, which in turn causes us to give up or give in and revert to our old lifestyle and unhealthy habits. So trade unhealthy choices for healthy options. For example, if you are drinking regular soda, then step down to diet soda. If you are already drinking diet soda, then evaluate how many a day you are drinking and start reducing the number of diet sodas you drink a day. Set a goal to consume only one diet soda a day by the end of twenty-one days. Drink water instead.

## Tip 4:

Turn off the TV unless you are exercising. This will be a stretch for some, but remember, twenty-one days and it will become life changing. We earn good health by cultivating healthy habits. Persistence will pay off. Be willing to remove distractions to speed up your success.

## Tip 5:

Reduce the number of times you eat out each week and incorporate new healthy habits into the process. Avoid fried food as much as possible. Split the restaurant meal with a friend or co-worker. Get a kids' meal instead of the adult version. Avoid coffee shops, vending machines, and convenience stores as much as possible. Most are full of unhealthy choices and too much of a temptation for your new lifestyle. Think moderation and pay attention to what you eat during the day.

## Tip 6:

Set an appointment with yourself for planning weekly meals and exercise. We set appointments for everything else in our lives. So put this daily and weekly schedule in your day timer. It is worth the time and effort.

**Tip 7:**

Consult your doctor and know your numbers before you start a health and fitness program. BMI, body fat, blood pressure, cholesterol, and LDL numbers are more important numbers than the numbers on the scale. Add a multivitamin to your daily plan. Women should also add a 1200 mg. calcium citrate supplement as well.

But don't forget the bottom line: The key to successful weight loss is a commitment to making permanent changes in your diet and exercise habits.

I would love to hear from you. I am also available to speak at group meetings, events, or conduct seminars. For products, a list of services, additional help, or information, please contact Joyce Ainsworth at **glenna@netdoor.com**

Your life change is a journey and the changes you make <u>today</u> will impact your tomorrows.

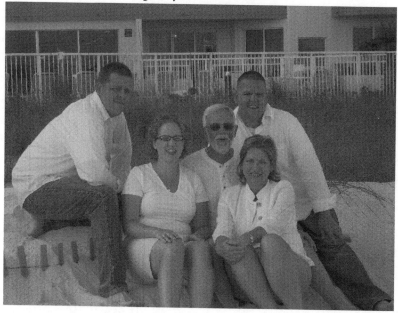

Life Change brings Joy!

# Positive Affirmations
## Change Your Thoughts Daily
## With Affirmations from God's Word

I am beautiful, capable, and lovable.
I am valuable.
I love myself unconditionally and nurture myself in every way.
I am unique, the apple of God's eye.

I am a child of God.
I love people and show love, warmth, and friendship to all.
I am healed of all my childhood wounds, and I hold no account of wrong done to me.
I can be honest with others and myself.
All of my relationships are based on integrity and respect.

I am intelligent and have great creativity.
I can concentrate easily.
I can analyze and solve problems.
I learn quickly and have an excellent memory.
I have the mind of Christ.
I can make decisions with confidence.

I am diligent, faithful, and have a spirit of excellence.
Whatever I put my hand to will prosper.
God always causes me to triumph in Christ.
I let go of things I cannot control.
I have the courage to change the things I should change, the serenity to accept the things I cannot change, and the wisdom to know the difference.
I have no need to control people or situations.
I am controlled by the Holy Spirit.

I am a success.

I can do anything I put my mind to.

I can do all things through Christ, who strengthens me.

I see each day as a new and positive adventure.

I give thanks in all things.

I express my potential more and more each day.

I see problems as exciting challenges that cause me to grow stronger and stronger in my faith.

✳ I visualize myself as the person God wants me to be.

I see myself achieving my goals and fulfilling God's purpose for my life.

I live every day with passion and power.

I feel strong, excited, passionate, and powerful.

I feel tremendous confidence.

I have all the abilities I need to succeed.

Every cell in my body vibrates with health, healing, vitality, and love.

I am healthy and strong and filled with vitality.

Jesus took every sickness and every disease away from me.

I awaken each day feeling healthy and alive with energy.

Any tension I feel is simply a signal to relax, release, and let go.

I always have more than enough energy to do all I want to do.

All that I am, I derive from Jesus.

He is always in my thoughts, and I pray without ceasing.

Jesus is my strength, my joy, my peace.

He is with me wherever I go, and He promised never to leave me or forsake me.

I surrender my life to Jesus Christ.
I have a wonderful, fulfilling relationship with Jesus.
I trust my conscience, which is led by the Holy Spirit.
I feel God's presence at all times.

I walk in the fruit of the Spirit of love, joy, peace, patience, goodness, gentleness, faith, meekness, and self-control.
I am sustained by the love of Christ.
The peace of God rests upon me.

I do not worry about anything.
In everything, I give thanks to God and give my cares to Him.
The peace that passes understanding guards my heart and mind, and I remain calm no matter what happens around me.

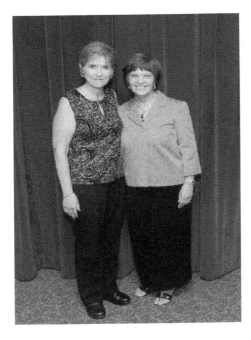

Joyce with Carole Lewis

# Sprint to the Finish

## Lose Those Last Few Stubborn Pounds

This section of the book has been designed to assist you in completing your journey to goal weight.

At this point I feel your frustration; I sense it even as I write this. You have tried everything. Nothing seems to work and you want to quit. Not this time. These final few pounds seem to be the hardest to lose, so gear up, get ready, and let's head to the finish line, but remember, this will only work if you do it. Just do it!

Let's take a good, hard look at your plan and identify some needed actions. Let me first remind you, for this to work, you have to do a complete evaluation of your whole program including food, tracking, and exercising programs. Now be honest with yourself. The final distance to the finish line depends on your honesty.

**Action 1:** The first action is to pull out your copy of the 21-Day Jump Start Plan and review the seven steps to preparation. Go back and make sure those steps are still relevant and active as part of your life change process. Tough situations call for tough measures, and you do not want anything to hold you back from making goal weight. Those seven steps of preparation were designed to set your environment up for success.

This is a time for re-establishing clear priorities to guide your steps and actions.

**Action 2:** Seek help and advice from a professional. At this point in my plan I consulted with a registered nutritionist. She had experience with individuals that had a history of obesity. She helped me re-focus on the important items at hand. She asked the hard questions and gave me an unbiased opinion about what needed to be done to accomplish my goal. She evaluated all my medical numbers and helped me understand where I needed to be and why. She evaluated my BMI, body fat, weight, blood pressure, thyroid, potassium, and other important numbers. She created a complete evaluation of my current plan and guided me to a few options to help me get to the finish line.

It is important to know and understand all these numbers; not just the number on the scale. She helped me realize the importance of my body fat and BMI and helped me analyze my food and fitness plans to reach the weight I wanted. She helped me decide if my goal weight was realistic, obtainable, and sustainable.

I challenge you to seek out expert advice, perhaps a dietician, nutritionist, personal trainer, life coach, or a combination of professional guidance. It will be money well spent. You cannot put a price tag on good health. Let's face it; most of us have spent a small fortune on "diet" aids through the years. Seeking professional guidance and advice are critical for your success.

**Action 3**: Re-establish your personal goal and make a plan. Avoid the rebellion mentality. After I met with the nutritionist I got mad. I complained about how life is not fair. My attitude was a guaranteed "plan" killer. Somehow, I expected the last ten pounds to be easy.

If you do not finish the race, you will once again be in bondage to food. Guilt, condemnation, isolation, and anger can derail you and produce failure. Bad habits have a way of pushing back into your life when you stop setting goals. God has a bigger plan than you can see. Remember, He wants us to trust Him for the finish while we do our part. We still have to do our part.

I started this journey because I had a desperate need to lose weight. I really had no other agenda at the time, but the Lord's plan included more than losing weight. Others are watching me. They will be watching and listening to you, too. They will model what we model.

Develop a never-quit mentality and a warrior mindset. There is no surrender or failure in the warrior code. Though none goes with you, determine there will be no turning back. If the scales never move downward again, there still can be no turning back. You're in until the end. Long-term and lasting life change is and should be your personal goal.

I determined going back to being overweight would never again be an option.

**Action 4:** Re-evaluate your accountability plan and build a team or a new team. Many of us are reluctant to include others in our journey. Accountability is a key component to success. You may need more than one person in this area. You may need a team. These accountability partners will help you with weighing in weekly, tracking food daily, and keeping up with your exercise plan. Building a team of accountability has three key elements: knowledge, practice, and coaching.

A. Knowledge: Attend a group. At FP4H, we study the Bible, memorize scripture, and pray for each other. Being part of the group allows me to establish relationships with other people who were encountering and experiencing the same life change difficulties. A regular and structured group offers help and support. Something is better than nothing, but face-to-face groups are the best option.

B. Practice: Keep running the race. Keep working on your food and exercise plans. Keep hanging out with others that are as concerned and conscious as you are. Allow another person to review your food plan and suggest big or small changes. Change often adds up to big results. Begin to practice life change with people who are as focused as you are on making great choices for real and lasting change.

The other day I went to a Subway with a group of friends. My friends went through the line and when I got to the register, I asked if anyone wanted a cookie. The whole group stopped to stare at me. Together they said, "No one sitting at our table is eating cookies today."

I got the message and refused a cookie as well. Had I been eating with a group who were all having cookies, I would have had a cookie, too. You get the picture? Friends and acquaintances can sabotage your success. So keep hanging out with like-minded people and continue to practice real and lasting life change.

C. Coaching: At times, we all need a coach or pacer. We need someone to help us along in the process of life change, someone who is willing to walk alongside us, encourage us, direct us, and correct us. That is what FP4H has been for me— my coach. It takes a huge act of courage to be willing to be vulnerable enough to allow someone into our lives to see the good, the bad, and the ugly. When we do, we see results. Practicing the principals of the life change process ensures success. Accountability is a key component. Be honest. It may be time to find a new coach for the completion of your journey.

**Action 5:** Re-evaluate your food and exercise plans. Sometimes finishing well requires adjustments in your food balance each day. I started eating different vegetables and different meats. I changed the type of snacks I ate. I had developed a habit of eating the same things repeatedly, so when I made adjustments, I shook up my metabolism. I measured and weighed my food more carefully. I only ate out of my portion control plate, tracked my food, and exercised with a new determination. You may need to revert to the same tactics you used when you began your journey. Be truthful about the size of your portions and the calorie count. Record food and exercise in a journal or on a tracking website honestly. If you cheat, you are only cheating yourself.

I adjusted my exercise plan, too. For example, I added a twenty-minute flexibility DVD to my fitness program each day and added additional abdominal crunches. I split my plan and exercised both morning and evening. I kept my body guessing about what would be next.

You could add yoga to your plan or water aerobics. Or how about a spin class? It could be as simple as doing your exercise in the morning instead of at night or vice versa. Be proactive and make some changes every few weeks until you make your goal weight. The real key is to make it fun and interesting, but don't expect it to be easy. Finishing is worth the extra effort.

Adjusting my food and exercise plan was a critical key to finally losing those last few pounds. Shaking up the body's metabolism can produce needed results.

**Action 6:** Re-commit to finish your journey. Give focused attention to the finish. Consistent obedience to the life change process must become a way of life permanently. To be obedient from the heart means to give yourself fully to God, to love Him with all your heart, with all your soul, and with all your mind.

Most of the time my effort to be consistently obedient would be considered half-hearted at best. On top of that, I expected to be blessed and rewarded for my half-hearted effort. Let's be honest. We often choose poorly in our food plan and eat things we know are not good choices. We avoid exercise. We don't take time to pray or plan our meals for the week, and then we are upset when there is no weight loss. We expect success for our half-hearted effort. Life change only happens when we focus on the finish and sprint to the end.

Identify what or who is holding you back, and regardless of your past success or failure, re-focus on the finish.

I made sacrifices of time and some activities that I loved so I could finish. It was and is worth the sacrifice and extra effort.

**Action 7**: Share the vision of victory with others. Have a victory party to celebrate when you reach your goal weight. Don't let food be the focus of the party. Go shopping for some new clothes. Clean out your closet. Donate or give away all those big clothes. If you really believe you are not going back, you don't need them. Continue to do the things that have brought you to the finish line. Set a new personal goal to help you stay on track for permanent life change. Then make a commitment to help someone else finish. Teach a fitness or FP4H class, join an online group, sign up for a 5K, half marathon, a marathon, or join a running group. Don't quit. Keep practicing your food and exercise plans. Keep them on your calendar or day timer. Develop a fool-proof maintenance plan. Become a Promised Land dweller, not a visitor.

You can do this! The finish line is possible and worth every ounce of effort you make. Don't give up! Focus on your Finish Line.

I'll see you at the Finish Line!

# What to Avoid as We Sprint to the Final Finish

**Fear:** Fear is a universal force that leads us to hide. (It started back in the Garden of Eden.) If we are going to experience freedom from fear, we must "faith" our fear. Try a replacement policy. Replace lies with the truth of God's Word. "There is no fear in love. But perfect love drives out fear, because fear has to do with punishment. The one who fears is not made perfect in love. We love because he first loved us" (1 John 4:18-19 NIV). God is on your side and by your side. "Who shall separate us from the love of Christ? Shall trouble or hardship or persecution or famine or nakedness or danger or sword? No, in all these things we are more than conquerors through him who loved us" (Romans 8:35, 37 NIV).

**Frustration:** Don't let the interruptions of life cause you to become frustrated. Plan and prepare for obstacles in all areas. Good intentions do not get the job done. Life change and finishing well should become priorities. Recall your purpose; rely on His power; rejoice as you persevere.

"Let us not become weary in doing good, for at the proper time we will reap a harvest if we do not give up" (Galatians 6:9 NIV).

**Failure:** When you don't see results, discouragement can hold you back. Keep pressing forward. Press into our Savior and allow Him to be your power source. You can stand in victory because He has paid the price.

"But thanks be to God. He gives us the victory through our Lord Jesus Christ. Therefore, my dear brothers and sisters, stand firm. Let nothing move you. Always give yourselves fully to the work of the Lord, because you know that your labor in the Lord is not in vain" (1 Corinthians 15:57-58 NIV).

Food has been a coping mechanism for a long time for so many of us. Now is the time to identify what we have tried to cope with. If you and I implement the tools in this book we can and will find success. We have to lose the failure mentality. God's Word says God wants us to get past our failures and mistakes, past the guilt, past the discouragement, and past the despair. You can make it this time. Trust Him! God is able. God is up to great things in your life and my life. Amazing things and yes he is a God that cares for you and me.

When you cross the finish line, we can all say the words of Paul together:
"I have fought the good fight, I have finished the race, I have kept the faith" (2 Timothy 4:7 NIV).

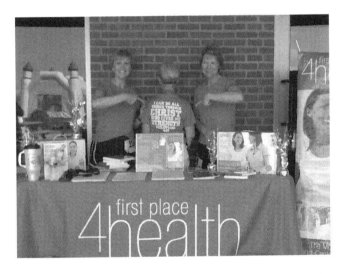

**Yes!**
**We can do all things through Christ who gives us strength**

# Healthy Food and Exercise Tips That Really Work

This section is designed to offer some extra tips on food and exercise. This is not an exhaustive list, simply some suggestions that might help in your personal journey. These ideas and tips are things that made a big difference for me.

## Tips on Food

**Have a healthy breakfast.** It is the most important meal of the day.

1. Eat healthy cereal. Top a high-fiber cereal with a sprinkle of granola, bananas, and low-fat milk or yogurt. This provides good fiber and protein plus calcium and potassium.

2. Eat berries with low-fat Greek yogurt with a drizzle of honey and a sprinkle of sliced almonds. These foods are high in protein which can help you feel full longer.

3. Choose nutrition to go. Smoothies are another smart choice when made with low-fat Greek yogurt and berries. Yogurt smoothies are high in protein, dairy, and volume. A smoothie is also portable if you're in a hurry. Pre-made wraps with ham and cheese or peanut butter are also good on-the-go choices.

4. Warm is always a good choice. Microwave one-quarter cup each of instant oatmeal and coarse wheat bran with a cup of milk (skim or 1 percent). Served with berries and a little maple syrup, it's the perfect start to the day. Or you could try an oatmeal soufflé (serving of oatmeal with one egg stirred in with a half cup of almond milk and microwave for a minute and a half) for a great breakfast choice. Serve with a little fresh fruit and yogurt and it is fabulous!

5. Don't skip on eggs. Scrambled egg – one whole egg and one egg white – along with a piece of whole wheat toast, lightly buttered with some fruit on the side, is a high-protein, high-volume combination. Breakfast burritos can spice up your morning meal. Try a scrambled egg, whole wheat (for extra fiber) wrap along with some salsa, low-fat sour cream or no fat plain Greek yogurt, and a sprinkle of cheese. Turkey bacon is another great option. Low sodium of course.

6. Try cottage cheese. Mixed with fruit or nuts, cottage cheese is a good breakfast choice high in protein plus it will help your calcium intake.

7. Think vegetables for breakfast. You can enjoy veggies with breakfast by adding them to eggs. Stir in some lightly steamed vegetables like broccoli or spinach with your scrambled egg. Add a little turkey bacon or place in a whole wheat wrap.

8. Use whole grains. Whole grain English muffins with peanut butter or another nut butter and sliced fruit, such as apples or pears, along with a glass of low-fat milk, can be filling while providing protein and calcium.

**Eat a variety of nutrient-rich foods.** You need more than forty different nutrients for good health, and no single food supplies them all. Your daily food selection should include bread and other whole-grain products, fruits, vegetables, dairy products, meat, poultry, fish, and other protein foods. Determine how much of each item by your calorie needs.

**Eat regular meals.** Skipping meals can lead to out-of-control hunger, often resulting in overeating. When you're very hungry, it's also tempting to forget about good nutrition. Snacking between meals can help curb hunger, but don't eat so much that your snack becomes an entire meal.

**Snacks are a needed part of a great food plan.** If you choose the right kind, snacks can be great healthy options. The list below offers between-meal bites that will help you stay satisfied. Look for snacks that contain protein, fiber, calcium, or antioxidants to keep your body at its best. The key is to have snacks that fend off a craving without a lot of added fat, sugar, or calories. No matter what you choose, try to choose well. Making good choices will make a difference. Make sure you plan two to three snacks a day. Several snacks a day keep the body fueled, and fat burning becomes more efficient.

1. Snacks should be less than 200 calories (even for men). Some suggestions: protein bar, peanut butter and crackers, Kashi granola bar, or Kellogg's Fiber One bar.

   Caution: The main thing to remember on snacks is to avoid high sugar or high fat items. Read the labels even on protein bars and granola bars. Some brands are packed with sugar and fat. Find a good quality food to have as a snack, but try to make sure it is a good protein choice and contains some quality carbohydrates.

2. Cheese sticks are a great option and easy to take along.

3. Nuts are another great option, but remember the best way to do these is pre-bag or buy in the 100-calorie packs. This makes a great choice, but no snacking right out of the can of large-volume items like nuts. Also, try the cocoa roasted almonds.

4. Nabisco 100 percent whole grain Fig Newtons, one-pound bag. Fig Newtons have gone whole grain. Two cookies have 110 calories, 2 g. fat, 0 g. saturated fat, 1 g. protein, 2 g. fiber, and 12 g. sugar (some of which comes from the figs).

5. Healthy Choice fudge bars, six bars per box. Per bar: 80 calories, 1.5 g. fat, 1 g. saturated fat, 3 g. protein, 4 g. fiber, 4 g. sugars, and 3 g. sugar alcohols.
Skinny Cow chocolate truffle bars, six bars per box. Per bar: 100 calories, 2.5 g. fat, 1.5 g. saturated fat, 3 g. protein, 3 g. fiber, 12 g. sugars, and 0 g. sugar alcohols.

6. Kellogg's cracker chips or Triscuits are both great snack choices. There are many fancy crackers on the shelf, but one of the best is an oldie but goodie, reduced-fat Triscuits. Some of the newer crackers are either high in fat and saturated fat, or low in fiber (even some types that sound like they'd have plenty of fiber). Learn to read those food labels.

7. Popcorn. Orville Redenbacher's Smart Pop, three bags per box. Per 3 tablespoons un-popped: 120 calories, 2 g. fat, 0.5 g. saturated fat, 4 g. protein, 4 g. fiber, and 240 mg. sodium. Smart Balance light butter popcorn (no diacetyl added), three bags per box. Per 2 tablespoons un-popped: 120 calories, 4.5 g. fat, 1.5 g. saturated fat, 3 g. protein, 4 g. fiber, and 290 mg. sodium.

8. Fresh fruit. Always a great option and always in season. Look for variety and try different fruits. Fresh fruit is always a quality option.

**Avoid high fat foods.** Avoid all fried foods. Avoid sugary foods with no real value for the body. Focus on high quality foods not high fat and calories.

**Try some chocolate peanut butter.** This is one of my favorite goodies. It makes a great pre-work out snack, is good at breakfast, snack, lunch, or dinner. It is a high quality food and gives that little chocolate fix without empty calories or bad fats. I spread a small amount on a low-fat whole grain wrap.

**Hummus is another great food I have discovered.** There are lots of varieties on the market. It can be used by itself or in combination with a small amount of salsa to create a spread for sandwiches, a base for dips, and can be added to chicken or turkey salad. Use hummus as a substitute for mayonnaise.

**Drink plenty of water and avoid sodas** and carbonated drinks as much as possible, including the diet kind. Once you get use to drinking water, your body will crave it.

**Do not skip meals.** Do not save foods from one meal to the next. Focus on balance in all meals. Focus on variety and quality in all your food choices throughout the day. Quality food in proper quantity guarantees results that are life-changing.

**Add a multivitamin** to your daily plan and for women a 1200 mg. calcium citrate supplement. I am not a big advocate of supplements, but a good multivitamin is important for everyone.

**Learn to eat with a purpose** and learn to manage your food choices. Food has no power over us unless we allow it. Dieting usually triggers the starvation reflex, so eating small meals frequently burns more calories.

**Find foods with moderate or lower calorie content** that make you feel satisfied. Never diet again! Learn to change your mind about food. To truly be successful you must monitor calorie and nutritional intake.

**Gain control over your intake of calories** by tracking your food. There are many great websites and tools to help track your food. Some suggestions are included in this book under the helpful websites and tools page.

This is not an exhaustive list but just some simple helpful tips I have learned along the way in my own personal journey. There are no good or bad foods. All food is permissible for me, but not all food should have a prominent place in my food plan. The best place to begin is to make a list of foods you really like and figure out a way to put them in your plan. Moderation, not deprivation, is going to be the real key to your success.

# Exercise Tips

**The only real requirement is to start.**

- **You deserve time to exercise.** We are better at other things if we take time to exercise. Make an appointment on your calendar for exercise. When exercising at the right level of effort the body, mind, and spirit come together to produce a feeling of great satisfaction. Exercise can be restorative and refreshing. The stress release from exercise is immediate and empowering. The real key is to have patience and don't give up. And don't forget to have some fun!

- **Ten-minute segments of exercise** throughout the day have helped me and will help anyone, especially on those long workdays. The American Heart Association suggests three to four workouts of ten minutes each, spread throughout your day. In the beginning, when longer workouts scared me, I began with shorter exercise times. Let's face it, the bigger you are the harder it is to get started with exercise, so break it up, but do something. I didn't want to think about doing anything for 30 minutes or an hour, but ten minutes was doable.

- **Mix it up.** Be sure to cross-train. Try to change up your daily workout. Watch one of your favorite TV shows and do strength training moves during the commercial breaks. Or try lunges, squats, and crunches. Remember, mix it up. Giving yourself mini, achievable health goals produces success. Mix it up in whatever you do. Fun is the key to continuing.

- **Change your scenery.** Workouts can get a little boring, so trade the treadmill for some new terrain and explore a great path in your neighborhood. Go for a long hike or a swim. A new environment can breathe fresh air into your routine. Change keeps your body guessing. Try different activities if you are a "gym junkie." Simply trying different machines or weights can help keep it interesting.

- **Do not use food as a reward.** Rewards are very important when it comes to an exercise program and in some cases can be crucial. Provide rewards that will keep you motivated and on track to your goals. New shoes or clothes, a massage, or a special trip to an event that you want to go to is much better than a food reward.

- **Leave the magazine at the house.** It might seem like a great way to keep yourself entertained during a workout, but if you can read captions in a magazine, chances are you're not pushing yourself hard enough. If you really feel a need to read, try downloading a podcast or listening to an audio book. The key is to make your workout count.

- **Buddy up.** I could not make it without my friends. Working out together is a great way to stick with a fitness routine. Meet each other for a run in the morning or take an aerobics class before or after work. Just make sure you partner with a pal you can count on to push you and help you reach your goals, not one that will be your partner in the crime of not following through.

- **Change gets your metabolism going.** Change up your workouts with a little high-intensity strength training. Increase the weight, reps and/or sets you lift (and decrease the amount you rest in between), and you'll start to see some sculpted, lean muscles. You will keep your metabolism humming post-workout. Also break it up. Break up the monotony by putting a set of abdominal crunches in between each set of your weight-training routines. Since you never have a chance to sit still and cool off, you'll keep your heart rate up and burn more calories and body fat.

- **It is important to dress for success.** Comfort above all else counts when it comes to shoes and clothes for exercising. Before you start any kind of exercise routine make sure your body is well supported. This means comfortable shoes of a good quality, high quality and supportive underwear (a strong sports bra for women), and breathable fabrics in shorts and shirts. You can focus on achieving better results instead of uncomfortable-fitting clothing if good choices are made ahead of time. Remember, to be successful at real life change we must have the right tools.

- **Another great tool for exercise** is a good step counter and/or heart rate monitor. I never exercise without my polar heart rate monitor; it keeps track of every calorie burned.

- **Music** has an amazing power to pump us up and get us going. Rather than relying on others to get you through a workout, organize some high-energy and uplifting songs on an iPod or MP3 player. Put your favorite songs at the beginning, middle, and toward the end to motivate you. Change it up every week by adding new songs or switching MP3 players with a friend. Music is a great motivator.

- **Have patience.** It took years to accumulate fat and it is really best to burn it off gradually. The key is to keep it off forever from this point on. The goal is to establish a positive relationship with exercise. We want to learn to love exercise.

- **Chaffing issues.** During warm weather or for larger people who exercise regularly, chaffing can be a problem. We have areas where clothing or body parts produce wear on other body parts. Reducing the friction in those areas will reduce the irritation. You can reduce friction and aggravation by using Vaseline and exercise products like Body Glide. Compression tights (these are shorts made of Lycra) have reduced chaffing between the legs dramatically. I still wear compression shorts for my workouts; it just makes good sense to me.

- **Excess skin:** Use girdles, spandex, or knee–to-chest body suits to help keep excess skin from getting in the way. Also make sure you dry off properly and shower right after a workout, walk, or run. Excess skin and moisture are a prime habitat for ulcers, skin rashes, and yeast infections.

- **Set doable short-term goals for yourself.** Once you reach that goal, immediately set another one. Also helping others train for a goal is motivating for you. You can help others while still helping yourself.

- **Don't quit.** Never give up on yourself. Exercise is the key to creating your fat-burning furnace. Exercise can and will make you feel better physically, mentally and emotionally. Exercise is a critical component to your life change process. If you fall off the exercise wagon, dust yourself off and start over. It is only considered failure if you don't get back up. So get back up and back on track.

Exercise was and still is a critical component to my life change process. I urge you to seek medical advice and get a wellness work-up before starting any exercise program. Always be willing to seek professional help. Adults who exercise are positive role models, and mothers who exercise are the most powerful role models to their own children. So lead by example. We need to be positive role models spiritually, physically, mentally, and emotionally for our children and others. The right attitude about food and exercise are learned behaviors. Kids who exercise have increased energy, improved attitude, more motivation, less stress, and do better in school academically. Kids who exercise develop a positive attitude about themselves and about life in general. Healthier kids become happier kids. What a great combination, and this fact alone should motivate us to learn to love exercise and pass it on.

What is stopping you? Whatever it is, it is time to let it go, move forward, and see the truth and power in exercise. No more excuses. Evidence is growing that exercise brings quality and longevity to your life and relationships. It will also bring to you better health mentally, emotionally, physically, and spiritually. Exercise is life changing!

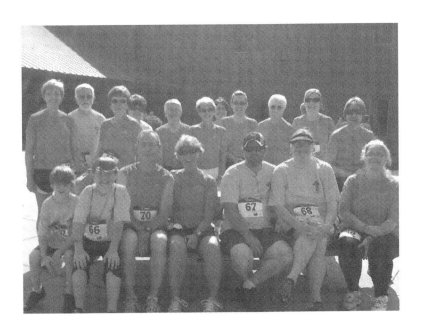

Team in training

Change Your Mind!
Change Your Body! Change Your Life!

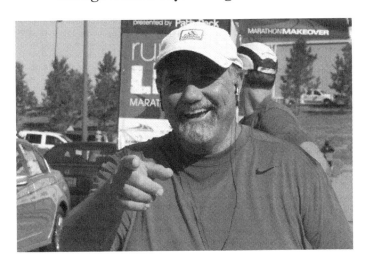

# 6 Week Study Guide

## Food, Freedom and Finish Lines!

This study guide has been designed to guide you and your small group through a deeper study of the book, *"Food, Freedom and Finish Lines"*. Group gatherings of many kinds will benefit from this study. It is designed to be experienced in a setting such as a Bible study group, First Place 4 Health group, or any small group where learning how to become and stay healthy by losing weight and making lifestyle changes are the goal. This study utilizes all the tools for success that are within the book and will guide you through the process of pin pointing specific areas of needed change whether that change is physical, mental, emotional or spiritual. Change will never be easy but the long term benefits will be out of this world.

### Materials Needed
In addition to bringing a Bible to group discussions, each participant should have his/her own study guide along with a copy of Food, Freedom & Finish Lines!

### Format
This Study Guide is suggested and arranged for a six-week study, where each week two chapters of the book, Food, Freedom & Finish Lines, are covered, except for the last week in which just one chapter is studied. Each day you will have a reading assignment, a positive affirmation to speak out loud which in itself will be life changing over the course of this study; questions to answer and ponder on and yes answers. We want to encourage you to share within your small group and each day closes with a food for thought segment. All components are designed to help you get the very most out of this study guide.

*We also want to note that this study guide could easily be expanded to a 12 week study by only using one chapter of the book each week.

### Timing
Length of time for this study is 25-30 minutes, depending on the size of the group and participation of members. Personal at home preparation for the class time should take about 15 minutes per day

## Special Acknowledgment

I want to take a moment just to mention and personally thank June Chapko for her invaluable help with this study guide. After many requests from FP4H Leaders all over the country for a study guide to go along with Food, Freedom and Finish Lines, I sensed in my spirit that this was a needed addition to my book and would have the potential to help many find a new level of help, hope and healing. I shared my thoughts and vision with my trusted and dear friend June and she began to assist me in birthing the study guide.

With June's invaluable help and by the Lord's direction the study guide is better than I could have envisioned on my own. Special thanks to June Chapko for her help in writing and editing this project. May the Lord Bless you June for your gifted service on this study guide.

## Personal Reflection by Joyce:

God has a way of marking some dates on our hearts that become unforgettable. For me it happened when I was 12 years old on a Sunday night at Highland Baptist Church in Crystal Springs, MS, on the back pew. The message that night spoke to me and in that moment I knew I had no "hope". I knew about Jesus (head knowledge) but I did not know Jesus (heart knowledge). I practically ran up the aisle so I could ask Jesus to come into my heart and forgive me for all my sin. It was the first time freedom whispered my name and my life changed that night; but I don't think at 12 I really understood the radical impact Jesus wanted to have on my whole person.

At the young age of 12 I found freedom but little did I know it was just the beginning of my life change journey. I had my "life Insurance" but at that point it was more a term policy instead of a whole life policy. At the age of 30 freedom once again whispered my name and in the stillness that followed I knew the longing in my heart was for more than just fire insurance. It was a deep longing for real freedom. That night in a small prayer room a broken and wounded mother of 3 cashed in that "term" policy with the Lord and bought into the "whole" life concept. At 12 I had made Him Savior but at 30 I "surrendered all" and made Him Lord. I held nothing back or so I thought; I was so tired of trying to do things my way.

Once again my life began to change but the Lord was not done. In the years that followed I began to realize there were areas in my life that still needed to be surrendered to the correction and care of the Savior. Jesus being the loving father that He is began to slowly tear down the walls I had so carefully built around my wounded and broken life. Jesus had come to give me freedom and his desire was for me to be free indeed.

What a journey the Lord has allowed me to travel over the last few years. He has radically and totally changed my life! Just in the last 6 or so years Jesus has changed my whole person by empowering me to lose a great deal of weight. WOW! He is in the weight loss business too! Food, Freedom and Finish Lines was another step in the process.

Now we have added the study guide and still Jesus continues to radically change my life even today. I have come to realize he does not just want to be part of my life. He wants to **BE MY LIFE.**

*John 10:10 says*
*The thief comes only to steal and kill and destroy; I came that they may have life and have it abundantly*

Faith to me is a journey; it is more a daily walk where I continually hear Freedom whisper my name. Jesus brings life out of death; he restores the broken and recovers the lost. He is Life!

### *LIFE (Living Intentionally ~ Focused Eternally)*

As you mark your journey through the pages of Food, Freedom and Finish Lines, remember this study guide has been created so that as you read my story the Lord might bring healing into many areas of your life. The Finish is not a onetime event but a daily process of life change.

**So drink deeply, be still and listen. Freedom is calling your name!**

*Faithfully His*
*Joyce*

# Week One: Where Are You?

**Word for the Week:**
Genesis 3:9 *"But the Lord God called to the man, "Where are you?"*

**Weekly Reading Assignment:** Chapters 1-2 in Food, Freedom & Finish Lines!

**Affirmation:** I am beautiful, capable, and lovable. I am valuable. I love myself unconditionally and nurture myself in every way. I am unique, the apple of God's eye.

## * Day 1: Evaluate

**Reading Assignment:** pp 13-16 in Food, Freedom & Finish Lines!

My entrance into the race of my life began with a photo and a question. You may recall how my daughter's wedding pictures prompted me to search for myself in the photos. It wasn't just the truth of my weight that was revealed in them. They led me to search deeper into the hidden places of bondage that kept me tethered to food.

Do you have a defining photo or event that declared itself as the search mode that caused you to ask yourself, "Where am I?" If so, describe it and allow yourself time to look deep into the hidden crevices of your soul. Where do you find yourself?

*Having to ask for extension for seat belt on plane + vacation pictures - How did I get here? Where am I?*

The smile I wore in the wedding pictures actually covered up the pain within my heart and soul. It covered up the hurtful words of childhood friends throwing them instead of sticks and stones. It covered my unbidden thoughts of unworthiness, shame and self-degradation.

Think about those past hurts that you may have endured outwardly, but you swallowed inwardly. Take some time and write about how you processed that hurt; withdrawal from others, turning to food, anger? Be specific: _Critical mother - verbally abusive. Led me_ _to a lifetime of perfectionism, self-doubt,_ _depression. Food became my comfort, so I ate_ _when I was sad, stressed, felt insecure, etc_ _Never felt "good enough"_

Read pp 18-19 in Food, Freedom & Finish Lines!

Physical hunger is the normal response to a legitimate need. We all experience the feelings of hunger, and eating is the natural response to that feeling. From a very young age, we are taught to eat, not because of a physical hunger but based on emotions. When a baby cries we give them a bottle, when a toddler falls down and has an injury we give them some ice cream. We also use food as a reward for all types of occasions.

Think and share about the times you have used food to meet an emotional hunger.
_I have used food when I was sad, feeling_ _insecure or unloved and when I was stressed_ _or angry_

We all have hungers deep within where no one can see. We seek comfort in wrong places. My silent hunger showed up in the eyes of an overweight mother in a wedding picture. My eyes cried out for help; I needed healing from a wounded heart and a fake smile. What place silently cries out in you? What or who are you seeking?
_My wounded heart - past insecurities, I am_ _seeking unconditional love and to feel "precious" -_ _which I know I have from God_

Turn to Genesis 3:8-9. Read and reflect on these verses and...
1. Why do you think God asked Adam and Eve, "Where are you?"
_He wanted them to think about what they had_ _done._

2. Insert your name before the question: ___Janice___, where are you? How would you answer?

_I am trying to break free from my past - to learn to listen to God's truths and not use food to numb my pain_

**Food for Thought:** Read Psalm 139: 23-24
It's important to remember that God knows every detail of your life. Think about His question again. If He knows where you are, why do you think He would ask you that question? Share your thoughts with God.

_I know Lord that you know everything about my life including my past hurts and insecurities. Help me Lord to look to you for your unconditional love and remember that I am your precious child._

## * Day 2: Searching

**Reading Assignment:** pp.17-18 in Food, Freedom & Finish Lines!

We are faced with so many opportunities to use food (rather than God), for comfort. Complete today's reading assignment. List some of the opportunities I mentioned, and then add some in which you have turned to.

_When we are happy, sad, stressed, tired, overworked or need a break — When we feel unappreciated or fall into the comparison trap_

There is nothing wrong with enjoying a good meal or celebrating special occasions where food is involved. It becomes a problem when we search for comfort, peace and fulfillment in food instead of searching for those things in God.

Read Isaiah 41:8-10
God chose Israel through Abraham because He wanted to! They were to represent God to the world. They failed to do what God wanted them to do. What does verse 10 say, and how does this verse encourage you?

_Do not fear, for I am with you ; do not be dismayed for I am your God, I will strengthen you and help you (when I am weak - He is strong)_

Read I John 1:9 and fill in the following blanks
If we __confess__ our __sins__, he is __faithful__ and __just__ and
will __forgive__ us our __sins__ and __purify__ us from all __unrighteousness.__

God is faithful, which is His character. God is just. Do you believe that? Search your heart and if necessary, confess any sin you feel is there. God wants to forgive because He loves you.

Read pp.18-19 in Food, Freedom & Finish Lines!

Nothing is more precious than a newborn baby. It doesn't matter whether they have no hair or a full head of it; if they are wrinkled or have smooth skin; what color eyes or skin they have; and it doesn't matter how much they weigh, preemie or full term. All babies are precious. How much more precious we are in God's sight. Our body make up doesn't matter when it comes to God seeing us as precious.

We, however, put up protective barriers to still the voice of pain. We have a hidden desire buried deep inside that cries out to be loved, cared for and protected. We want to be precious to someone. The barriers we erect when we are overweight keep others from getting close. We may even block access to our heart from God, the very One who can give us what we hope for.

Read Ephesians 1:18 and meditate on it for a while. Deep inside, we all want to have the hope that we will have victory through God. Now, look up the following Scriptures and write down the common thread found in each one.

Romans 8:23-25 __hope for what we do not yet have__
Ephesians 4:4 __one hope__
Colossians 1:5 __hope that is stored in heaven__
1Thessalonians 1:3 __hope in our Lord Jesus Christ__
1 Peter 3:15 __the hope that we have__

The hope we have is not some elusive butterfly we chase or a feeling of vagueness that everything will be bright and rosy in the future. Our Hope is the assurance that in Jesus Christ we have certain victory. He is our hope.

Read 1 John 5:4 reflect on it; then write it out here in your own words.

_As believers we have victory over the sins of_
_the world_

**Food for Thought:** The first chapter of Ephesians contains a list of the spiritual blessings you have in Christ. Read it through and jot down the ones that make you feel precious.

_chosen, blameless in His sight, adopted as His child,_
_redemption, forgiveness, wisdom, power of the_
_Holy Spirit_

## * Day 3: Change will Come

**Reading Assignment:** Read pp 20-21 in Food, Freedom & Finish Lines!

We know that God knows exactly where we are. We have spent the week evaluating, seeking and searching so that we know where we are. That is an important step. Yesterday, we spent time understanding how precious we are to God. Today we will take all that we've learned and face the truth. The truth is that God waits for you to cry out for help to the one and only great Healer, and ask Him to help you change.

Will change be easy? Of course not! But, it is possible! Are you willing to bring your struggles with food, eating and weight (or any other addiction) to Him in honest surrender?

Read Matthew 5:6 (ESV)
What does the word "satisfied" in this verse mean?

_Filled with the Holy Spirit_

When we hunger and thirst, seek and search after righteousness, after Jesus, we will be satisfied. We won't need to run to food, idols or any other thing to satisfy our hunger any longer.

Read Psalm 103:1-5 and record the benefits in the following verses:

Vs 3 _forgiveness, healing_

Vs 4 _redemption, love, compassion_

Vs 5 _satisfaction, renewal_

Which of these benefits do you desire in your life?

_Forgiveness, healing, satisfaction, renewal_

**Food for Thought:** Don't beat yourself up for not having enough will power to lose weight on your own. Come face to face with the Lord and allow Him to show you that allowing food to comfort you can be sin, and let that be your turning point, as it was mine. Is God whispering "freedom" to you now? Are you willing to change even though it won't be easy?

It could be the first prayer you need to pray is the same one I prayed. Lord I am not willing but make me willing. If this is the "truth "of where you really are just tell the Lord and He will hear your heart. He will enable you to make the changes needed. Trust Him to do the hard work but allow Him to show you the path to real and lasting freedom.

## * Day 4: Attitude Adjustment

**Reading Assignment:** pp 23-27 in Food, Freedom & Finish Lines!

**Affirmation:** I live every day with passion and power. I feel strong, excited, passionate and powerful. I feel tremendous confidence. I have all the abilities I need to succeed!

If our attitude is going to change it must begin in the mind. When we change the way we think, the way we act, the way we feel, and how we approach life, change will take place. Our Word for the Week explains that it's all in what we have our minds set upon; that is how we will live and how we will act, feel and approach life. If change is to take place in your life, you will need to look at your attitude and see what your mind is set upon. Place a check mark next to any of the following attitudes you may have now or had earlier in life. Then explain how it has affected you in the area of your weight.

- God doesn't care about this area of my life; He has more important things to deal with.
- ✓ I'm too old to make changes in my life; I'm too set in my ways.
- God made me this way and He loves me; why should I worry about my weight?
- I don't care what people think of me; they will just have to get over it.
- ✓ My physical limitations prevent me from exercising; that's why I'm overweight.
- ✓ It's in my genes. All my family is fat. I've accepted it.
- Other:
  _____
  _____
  _____

It is a proven fact that diets do not work; never have; never will. A diet only forces the body to do something that the mind has not agreed to do. That is one reason we never seem to be able to stick with a diet. The body might change, but the mind still wants those unhealthy habits it has been indulging in for so long. It craves the things it has been a slave to.

Read 2 Peter 2:17-19 and answer the following questions.

What is a man a slave to?
Whatever has mastered him
_____
_____

Read Ephesians 4:22-24 and spend time today meditating on these verses. Ask God to help you change your attitude and change your mind so that real and lasting change will come. This Scripture passage addresses three specific areas of life: the past, the present and the future. In regard to your former way of life, (the past), what specifically are you to do with it and why?

_Put off your old self - it was being_
_corrupted by its deceiptful desires_

Are you ready to do that? Who was in control in your former way of life? _myself_

The next part of the verse in Ephesians is present tense, being "made new," an ongoing renewal process. Life change isn't a one-time fix but a _repetitive_ Process (page 26). Today is the time to allow God to begin the process of changing your mind, attitude and heart about food. It's time to allow Him to peel away layers of negative self-talk and things that have you bound.

Are you willing to ask God to begin? Write a short prayer here and let Him know you are giving Him permission to come in and help you today.

_Lord, I surrender myself and my problems with_
_food and overeating to you. I ask you to come in_
_and take control of my choices and to change my way_
_of thinking_

The future part of this verse helps us look deep into the heart of God. He loves us. He wants us to be forever changed beginning on the inside and becoming more dependent upon Him for the power to change our mind, our body, our life. Fill in the blanks for verse 24. "and to put on the new self, _created_ to be like _God_ in true _righteousness_ and _holiness_ ."

**Food for Thought:** I knew that for me to be successful, really successful, at the weight-loss journey, it would require a lot of prayer time, daily Bible reading/study, and Scripture memorization.

Decide today that you will make these key elements of your relationship with Christ a priority, and be consistent in agreeing with God about His plan for you; not your plan, but His plan.

# * Day 5: God's Plans Work

**Reading Assignment:** page 28 in Food, Freedom & Finish Lines!

In my personal reflection I wondered if I could really make it to the finish line. Have you ever questioned that in your own life? Have you pondered in your heart the possibility of every reaching that seemingly elusive goal weight? I believe anyone who has struggled over and over with diets and weight loss schemes, has asked themselves that same question.

Share a time when you struggled with that question.

*Many times after trying to lose weight, only to gain it back plus some. Almost afraid to try again because of fear of failure (again)*

A discovery I made might also help you as we journey together with our weight issues. That discovery is this; Real change can only begin when we allow the truth of God's Word to make the transformation. When He became the center of my life, I found balance and learned to address my problems. I found that I had to become more dependent upon Him and less dependent upon Joyce, for the ability to transform my life. Are you ready to make that change?

*Yes!*

Read Philippians 4:13 and write it out here.

*I can do everything through him who gives me strength.*

That verse needs to be firmly set in your mind, memorized and meditated upon. You CAN do all things, but only if you do them through Christ. He is your strength giver! When the road is rocky, repeat that verse out loud, over and over until you believe that He really is the one giving you strength.

Christ is the source of all truth and when you allow Him to become the center of your life you will find balance, and you will learn to face those challenges and problems, including weight issues, and your life will be changed forever.

**Remember:** The day is coming when you can stand at the finish line and say:

*Job completed: Impossible is a lie! By the Power of Christ!*

**Food for Thought:** Lasting change will always start in the mind because we are made new in the attitudes of our minds. Think about some of the attitudes you have had in the past concerning food and exercise. Have you hung on to some of them? Write out the old attitudes and a new one using Scripture to replace it.

| Old Attitude | New Attitude |
|---|---|
| I can't do this | Philippians 4:13 |
| Arthritis makes exercise hard, painful | |
| I've failed so many times | |

**\* Day 6: Personal Evaluation**

**Reading Assignment:** pp 132-133 in Food, Freedom & Finish Lines!

If you desire real life change to happen and want to strengthen those areas of weakness in your life, you must be willing to face the truth and ask for help. You cannot change what you are unwilling to admit! You cannot stick your head in the sand and pretend everything is okay. Today, take the time to answer the questions on pages 132 and 133 concerning where you are in your journey. It doesn't matter whether you have a lot of weight to lose or if you are struggling to get those last few pounds off. You may even have some other type of bondage. By taking a personal evaluation, it will help you discover where you are and what changes you need to make to cross YOUR finish line.

**Food for Thought:** Once you complete the personal evaluation, take time to consider your answers. Review them, pray over them, lay them on the altar before the Lord and surrender them to His Lordship. Allow Him to bring true healing and comfort. Freedom is possible!

## * Day 7: Personal Evaluation Assessment – Fast Facts

**Reading Assignment:** pp 134-135 in Food, Freedom & Finish Lines!

If we do not acknowledge where we are, we cannot begin to change. Hopefully, you completed the Personal Evaluation honestly and are now aware of the areas of change that are needed. Today you will read and consider the following 5 fast facts that will help you move forward in your journey toward the finish line.

### Fact 1: Re-evaluate
Who did you ask to go over the evaluation with you? Did you consider all four areas (mental, emotional, spiritual and physical)?

_Brooke_ _____

_____

_____

### Fact 2: Re-establish
Have you established that your personal goal is doable and attainable? Do you have a plan for stopping poor and unhealthy habits from reappearing in your life?

_____

_____

_____

### Fact 3: Re-organize
Who is on your team of accountability? We need different people in different seasons and for different reasons. You must give your accountability partners permission to get in your business in all areas if you want to succeed and finish strong.

_____

_____

_____

## Fact 4: Re-vamp

Mix things up a bit from time to time. Move things around if necessary; eat different foods, plan different times for exercise, etc. Don't get in a rut! How do you plan to revamp your plan?

_Try new recipes - Keep menu ideas that I enjoyed - try new exercises_

## Fact 5: Re-commit

Will you commit today to complete your journey and take someone with you to the finish line!

**Food for Thought**: Think about today's fast facts and pray over them. Are there any you might struggle with? If so, ask God to help you. Write a prayer to the Lord here.

# Week Two: Surrendering

## Word for the Week:
*"Those who live according to the sinful nature have their minds set on what that nature desires; but those who live in accordance with the Spirit have their minds set on what the Spirit desires."*
Romans 8:5

**Affirmation:** I see problems as exciting challenges that cause me to grow stronger and stronger in my faith. I visualize myself as the person God wants me to be. I see myself achieving my goals and fulfilling God's purpose for my life.

**Weekly Reading Assignment:** Chapters 3-4 in Food, Freedom & Finish Lines!

## * Day 1: Standing at the Crossroads

**Reading Assignment** pp 31-33 in Food, Freedom & Finish Lines!

Have you experienced standing at a crossroad in your life and knew you would have to choose one way over another? Briefly explain your most recent crossroad experience.

*Deciding to join FP4H and commit to doing all parts of it*

Some crossroads are as simple as which route to take to work, or what outfit do I wear today. Others are more crucial such as who should I marry, what career do I choose, or will I accept Christ as my personal Savior. We encounter many such crossroads throughout our lives and our choice can be a pivotal circumstance that can change the course of our life-changing journey. Your choice to join a FP4H group, or stop smoking, or begin an exercise program, can be a decision that will completely change your life. The outcome of your choices will be either positive or negative and the consequences are certain.

Read Deuteronomy 30:11-19
The Israelites were at a crossroad and God made it very clear what the consequence would be for either choice. What were their choices and the consequence that would result?

| Choice | Consequence |
|---|---|
| Love the Lord, follow His commands - | the Lord will bless you |
| Disobedience, worshipping other gods | Destruction - you will not live long |

As you continue on this journey you will encounter crossroads of whether to follow the plan and new lifestyle or forsake this healthy journey you are traveling. It is good as you encounter a crossroad to go back and re-read this passage in Deuteronomy. We always have a choice because God gave us a free will. Before you surrender, there is always a crossroad.

In today's reading assignment you discovered an example of what forced surrender was, based on the old TV program, *The Roy Rogers Show*. Think about what brought you to the place where you realized that changing your eating habits was something you would have to do. Does it fit the example of forced surrender? Explain why or why not.

In the past I've had the attitude of forced surrender - would find many excuses - when my attitude is not right I cannot be successful

Willing surrender is represented by The *Andy Griffith Show* where the character Otis willingly surrenders and puts himself in the jail cell. The sheriff didn't force him or even coerce him. Both forced and willing surrender involve the body, attitude, emotions and mind, but the outcomes are different. Does your attitude fit the example of willing surrender? Explain

My attitude this time is willing surrender - to work with God, not against Him - to depend on His strength and not my own. To surrender daily

**Food for Thought**: Where are you in your crossroad decision? Have you surrendered forcibly or willingly? Or, are you still standing there trying to decide? Talk to God about it right now.

## * Day 2: Pressures and Challenges

**Reading Assignment:** pp 34-43 in Food, Freedom & Finish Lines!

I'm reminded of the little boy sitting in time out. He had been a bit rebellious and his mother told him he would have to sit there by himself and think about his behavior. He responded, "I'm sittin' down on the outside but I'm standin' up on the inside!" You may be thinking that you want to lose weight on the outside, but the old mind has not come to that place of agreement. God will teach you bit by bit along the way and as He controls your mind you will see results. Setting small, achievable goals is an important step in your journey. My first goal was to weigh less than 300 pounds. My first mile marker was going from 339 pounds to 299 pounds! Achieving that weight loss and with my new mindset, I knew I needed a long-term plan. I needed to pursue a healthy plan.

Look up the word "pursue" and write down the definition.

*To follow and try to catch or capture (someone or something) for usually a long distance or time.*

It is important to realize that your old plan of unhealthy eating is part of your past. What did your old plan look like?

*Eating whatever I wanted - whenever I wanted combined with periods of healthy eating. Inconsistent - lots of emotional eating.*

I found "pursue" means "to follow close upon (someone or something) in a persistent way." Pursuing something new means some kind of action and that frightens people who have failed in the past. But just as your old eating plan is of the past, so is that frightened mind pattern of failure.

Read Isaiah 43:18-19 and write what the Lord is saying.

*Do not dwell on the past - God is doing a new thing*

Allow the Lord to give you mile makers; short, realistic NEW goals. These will help you succeed daily as you develop a long-term plan that will change you mentally and physically; inside and outside.

You read in today's assignment about how I did not like any kind of healthy food and French fries and ice cream were my foods of choice. My fish choice (fish is healthy, right?), which I ate plenty of, was fried catfish. Can you remember some unhealthy food choices you convinced yourself were fairly healthy?

Salad with lots of toppings / added ingredients

Change isn't easy when we do it ourselves, and I wanted this to be easy! So I did what I had to do to be really successful. I asked God for a plan. He was faithful to give it to me and I named it my "Step Down Plan." It was simple; just make changes in small baby steps. Instead of going 'cold turkey,' I modified the way I thought about the changes I needed to make. For instance; being on a 'diet' always made me feel deprived, so I decided to never use the word diet again and even today I focus on making small changes that will help me change my lifestyle. So think of your plan as a **permanent** change. Not something you go on and go off of. This was how I "put on the new self," (Ephesians 4:24).

Small changes that were doable, step by step, is how I stepped down to a healthy weight goal. Are you willing to make similar changes as God renews your mind and you begin putting on the new self? Circle any of these following things that might help you step down (knowing you can step down further as you begin seeing results). Then jot down others that come to mind in the space provided.

- Drinking diet colas instead of regular sodas
- Changing from full fat milk to low fat milk
- Choose sugar free items instead of the ones that are laden with sugar
- Adding a healthy snack into my afternoon to keep me from over eating at dinner.

- Choosing a piece of fruit instead of high calorie or high fat desserts
- Choosing baked or grilled instead of fried foods
- Drink more water
- Eat a healthy breakfast
- Choose to have the child's meal instead of the "super size" when eating out

_____

_____

_____

**Food for Thought:** Prayerfully consider a "Step Down Plan" for yourself. Think about your weakest areas of eating healthy. Would you be willing to limit red meat to 3 days a week instead of 5, by replacing it with fish, poultry or vegetarian? Could you go from whole milk to 2% for two weeks, and then step down to 1%? How about exercise? If you're not exercising at all, could you walk around your back yard twice? Or go bike riding for 15 minutes? Maybe you do not have a regular quiet time; how about 5 or 10 minutes with the Lord each morning for one month just to say thanks for Him loving you? Write out your Step Down plan using one item for each area; physical, mental, emotional and spiritual.

Physical:
   ↑ walking time - add strength & flexibility exercises

Mental:
   Read affirmations daily

Emotional:
   Positive attitude - connect with others

Spiritual:
   Continue daily Bible reading / quiet time

Spend time in prayer about each of these and ask God to help you Step Down.

# * Day 3: Success Requires Training

**Reading Assignment:** Pages 45-47 in Food, Freedom & Finish Lines!

It doesn't matter what you are trying to achieve; if you want to succeed you must work at it and train for it. A high school diploma requires it. A new position at work wouldn't last long without it. Learning any skills in sports, trades or business puts training at the top of their prerequisites. Athletes put in many long, hard days of training in order to succeed and win.

There is a saying I saw somewhere and I wrote it down and keep it on my desk. It says "Don't practice until you get it right; Practice until you can't get it wrong". That is the kind of practice real life change takes. We keep doing it until it becomes second nature to us, and the new nature or our new self takes on life.

As you began this program, you were asked to set a goal for the session. What was the goal you put down?

_To lose 20 pounds_

_____

_____

Preparing and training go hand in hand. "If you fail to plan, you are planning to fail." You train yourself on how to eat healthier; how to think differently; what your body is capable of in the way of physical activity; and how you relate emotionally and spiritually. Then you practice. Training requires a plan. Practice perfects the plan. What is your action plan to achieve the goal you listed above?

_____

_____

_____

In the book of Nehemiah, we can learn some key points on how to succeed. On page 47 in Food, Freedom & Finish Lines! I listed the ones that made an impact on me. Read that and then turn to Nehemiah, scanning chapters 2-6 and see for yourself what Nehemiah did that helped him succeed in rebuilding the wall in just 52 days.

List some of your findings below.

_He prayed_ _He helped others_
_He planned/developed a strategy_ _He prayed for_
_He enlisted help_ _strength_

Now look back over chapter six and study chapter seven. Did Nehemiah have the full support of the people he served? Were they cheering him on to the finish line? What did they tell him?

_____

_____

_____

Nehemiah followed his plan. He did not quit! He focused on the work at hand and followed through with the rebuilding. You are in the process now of rebuilding your temple and you have a plan. Do not allow anything or anyone (including your old self), to deter you or cause you to quit. Trust the Lord. He will see you to the finish line just like he did for Nehemiah.

**Food for Thought:** The book of Nehemiah was about rebuilding the wall of a great city, but it was also about the spiritual renewal and rebuilding of a people's dependence on God. You are in God's training program and He wants you to keep going regardless of whether or not others support you or cheer for you.
God is your support and cheering section. Submit and surrender any rebellion or sin to Him and ask forgiveness.

_____

_____

_____

_____

If you are unsure of any in your life; ask Him to reveal any unconfessed sin to you He is on your team and wants to see you succeed.

# * Day 4: Success Story

**Reading Assignment:** pp 49-54 in Food, Freedom & Finish Lines!

In my book, Donna Conerly shares her success story. She says that "Real Life Change" began for her in January 2009 when she joined FP4H weighing 189 pounds. She is a person, a real person just like you, who had tried many things to lose weight in the past. She admits she was scared because in the past she had lost and gained, while adding extra weight with each gain. On page 52, she mentions that in between FP4H sessions she attended a class to help her not break the pace she had set for herself. What type of class was it? Circle the one you think she attended.

~Exercise class        ~Water aerobics        ~Walking group
   ~Accountability group        ~Zumba Class

If you circled Accountability group, you are correct. How do you think her attending this class helped her stay on track? Why?

_She had someone else to report to so it helped her to continue to follow the program_

Do you know someone you might be able to ask to hold you accountable? This works both ways, they help you and you help them. When you are accountable to others, what will that do to help you succeed?

_It will help me stay focused on my goals_

On page 53, Donna gives God credit for giving her the desire to make a life change rather than continue to live on a diet plan. She gives some reasons for her being successful. What are they?

_God gave her the desire to change her life (not be on a diet) She admitted her addiction to food. She asked God for help. She was consistent._

**Food for Thought:** Do you REALLY want to be successful at losing this weight or making some other kind of real life change rather than continuing the same vicious cycle you have in the past? Will you allow God to give you the desire to make real and lasting life change this time? Talk to Him now; write a prayer of thankfulness here in the space provided and be ready to act on what He tells you.

*Thank you Lord for my FP4H group and for all that I have learned so far. Help me to see this as a total life change so that I can become healthier and serve you more.*

## * Day 5: Rest

**Reading Assignment:** page 55 in Food, Freedom & Finish Lines!

Donna recognized that rest is super important toward achieving success. She mentions physical rest so that her body can run and perform at its best. But she also knows that we need time to rest, reflect and revive our spirits. To do that, we need to spend time with our Heavenly Father and draw close to Him. The obvious question is: Have you made Christ the center of your life by asking Him to be your personal Savior? It is simple; confess that you have sinned, ask Jesus to forgive you and tell Him you want Him to be the center of your life. He is waiting to hear from you. You might want to pray this prayer.

*Jesus, I know that I'm a sinner and I'm sorry. Please forgive me. I believe that You, God's only Son, took my sins to the cross and You died for me so that I would live with You one day in heaven, forever. Thank You, Lord, for dying for me. I want You to be the center of my life, my Savior. Come into my heart, dear Jesus. Amen.*

If you prayed this prayer for the first time and have accepted Jesus as your Savior, please tell others. Let your group leader or pastor know about your new life in Christ. They will celebrate with you and rejoice over you. If you already know Christ as your Savior, can you say that you find rest in Him? Rest from worry, pain, outer circumstances of life? If not, ask Him to give you His rest.

# * Day 6: Healthy Tips

On pages 158-159 there are some tips on food and exercise that might help you in your personal journey. They made a difference for me and I pray they will for you. Read the four tips on food and decide how you might incorporate some of them into your eating lifestyle. Then after each tip, write your thoughts about how you will use that tip. These tips encourage you to eat a healthy breakfast because it's the most important meal of the day.

1.  Eat healthy cereal. Make it high fiber and choose from the following toppings: A sprinkle of granola, bananas, and low-fat milk or yogurt. What makes this combination important?

    _High fiber, calcium, potassium, protein_

2.  Eat berries with low-fat Greek yogurt and add a drizzle of honey and a sprinkle of sliced almonds. What makes these foods important?

    _high protein - helps you feel full longer_

3.  Choose nutrition to go. Smoothies made with low-fat Greek yogurt and berries are high in protein, dairy and volume. What other foods make good on-the-go choices?

    _Premade wrap — fruit — breakfast cookies_

4.  Warm is always a good choice. On page 158 there are two suggestions you may want to try. Choose one and write down which you tried and what you think of it.

    _____

    _____

**Food for Thought:** Variety is the spice of life when it comes to balanced living. If you will incorporate the above tips into your daily menus, it will help you keep from feeling bored with meals. You will be much more successful at Life Change when you add variety into every aspect of your plan.

## * Day 7: Jump Start

**Reading Assignment:** pp. 140-141 in Food, Freedom & Finish Lines!

Read through the seven steps to preparing yourself for victory. Begin today working through the steps and make notes as you complete each one. Some steps are quick and easy while others will have to be done over time. The important thing is to begin! The following check list will help you get started.
Remember we practice being healthy!

Step 1: Be willing to have someone weigh you each week. Who will that person be? _First Place_

Step 2: Clean out your kitchen, including the refrigerator and pantry. Today you might start with one or two items. Which will you clean out? Where will you choose to start?

Step 3: Portion Control Plate. Do you have one? If not consider buying one. You can e-mail me at **glenna@netdoor.com**

Step 4: Accountability Partner. Find someone willing to hold you accountable in your eating and exercise plan. Who will it be?
_Brooke_

Step 5: Join a bible study or support group; preferably a FP4H group. If there isn't one in your area, contact me at **glenna@netdoor.com** or FP4H at **www.firstplace4Health.com** and we will help you find one. Do you have one?

Step 6: Learn to track your food. Do you have a food tracker? What kind?
_My Fitness Pal_

Step 7: Commit to a fitness program. What are you doing currently?

_Walking - with goal of 10,000 steps/day_

Yesterday we began with four tips toward eating healthier at breakfast. Remember; don't skip this most important meal of your day! Today we'll look at four more tips (page 159), for you to blend in with the others and round out your week of healthy breakfast.

5.  Don't skip on eggs. There are several suggestions given for healthy eating. Which one sounds like something you will try in the coming week?

    _____

6.  Try cottage cheese. Mix it with fruit or nuts and it becomes a breakfast high in protein plus some calcium. Can you think of other ways to use cottage cheese as a healthy breakfast choice?

    _____

7.  Breakfast Veggies! Add them to eggs. Try lightly steamed broccoli or spinach. Add tomatoes and onions to make a tasty omelet. Other veggie breakfast ideas?

    _mushroom omelet — tomato, avocado, egg sandwich_

8.  Use whole grains. Many choices here. How about whole grain English Muffins with peanut butter and sliced fruit? Add a glass of low-fat milk and you will have a filling breakfast with protein and calcium. What other nut-butters could you choose?

    _almond butter_

**Food for Thought:** You need more than forty different nutrients for good health and no single food supplies them all. Think variety every day. Stay within your calorie range and get your day off to a healthy start. Eating a healthy breakfast will kick start your day and your metabolism. It is a proven fact that a healthy breakfast in the morning helps your body become a fat burning machine the rest of the day. Don't skip breakfast.

# Week Three: Detours

**Word for the Week:** *Consecrate yourselves, for tomorrow the Lord will do amazing things among you."* Joshua 3:5

**Weekly Reading Assignment:** Chapters 5-6 in Food, Freedom & Finish Lines!

**Affirmation:** I have a wonderful, fulfilling relationship with Jesus. I trust my conscience, which is led by the Holy Spirit. I feel God's presence at all times.

Life comes with detours! Of course, that's probably not a surprise to you. You've most likely experienced many of them. This week we'll consider the many aspects of detours and how we handle them.

Some detours are unpleasant, while others may be beneficial or protective. Today, we will look at several types of detours and their meaning. You may see some of them as familiar or they may never have occurred to you as being a detour.

Our Word for the week encourages us that the Lord has some amazing things He wants to do among us. Some of them may require us to take a detour from the path we want to take versus the one the Lord has laid out for us. Let's take a deeper look at some of the warning signs and the detours we sometimes take in our health journey.

## * Day 1: Warning Signs

**Reading Assignment:** pp 57-70 in Food, Freedom & Finish Lines!

Have you experienced a time when you were chugging along the highway and suddenly without warning, detour signs appeared, shuffling you off one road onto another? You may have had no idea there was a problem ahead until those red signs glared at you, preventing you from continuing the path you had chosen to drive.

These warning signs might be to protect you from danger ahead due to an accident or construction. What do you do when this happens?

_Most of the time I fuss & complain_

Have you been given any advance warnings by God of a detour along your journey? Explain what it was and how it felt.

In your weight loss journey, God may choose to provide a detour for you to help you avoid temptation (see 1 Corinthians 10:13).

It's important to realize that you have the choice of observing and following the detour signs. If you ignore them, consequences are sure to come. Can you share a time when you ignored one of God's detour signs? Describe the consequences?

There are short and long detours, as well as some that seem like a desert experience, where we wander around like the Israelites. Look up the definition of detour in the dictionary and write one that might apply to your FP4H journey.

_A deviation from a direct course or the usual procedure, especially: a roundabout way temporarily replacing part of a route._
_Cambridge: route taken in order to avoid a particular problem or to do something special_

Read page 59 and answer the question: What is the common denominator for all detours? _pain_

What does it do?

_throws us off pace_

Emotional devastation can be a real detour. When we give in to pain and emotional detours, the consequences can be overwhelming. My cookie catastrophe cost me many tears and pain, but God knew where I was and even cookies after a tornado couldn't prevent Him from reaching down and loving me right where I was. But He didn't leave me there.

Can you think of a situation that caused you to turn back to food, only to regret it later? What emotions did you express and how did God use it to reach you?

_anger, depression → overeating_

**Food for Thought:** Read my personal reflection on page 64. Think about the suggestions I listed for training to prepare for detours. Which ones jump out at you?

_recover quickly to limit damage to obtaining goals_
_Be prepared_
_Don't quit! Choose to get back up._

Write out a prayer to the Lord asking Him to help you take only the detours he has for you and to avoid the ones of your own making.

_Lord, I ask for your help in changing my life and following the FP4H plan. Help me to recognize detours that you have for me and help me to learn what you are teaching me through them. Help me to avoid detours of my own making that can cause me to stumble in my journey._

* **Day 2: Dream Big**

**Reading Assignment:** pp 72-73 in Food, Freedom & Finish Lines!

Read the quote from Martin Luther King Jr. that he gave the day before he was assassinated (bottom of page 72 and top of page 73).

Can you relate any of what he said to your FP4H journey? Share in what way.

_If I stay focused on Christ He will help me reach my goal._

## Read Joel 2:28

Joel predicted that God's Spirit would be poured out on all people and they would be given equal access to God's power. It did indeed happen. It was fulfilled in the events of the day of Pentecost. Believers everywhere have the power of God within them. They have the power to dream big dreams.

What is your dream regarding your health and wellness?

_To be active, improve my BP, cholesterol and lower my BMI, have more energy_

Your dream may be hidden deep, as was mine. It may have been hindered by feelings of defeat and failure. Martin Luther King Jr. was a man not to be held back by these things. He was passionate about what he believed and that passion drove him to keep going around and through detours. What about you? Can you depend upon God's power, the Holy Spirit that is in you, to realize your dream?

**Food for Thought:** Think about your dream and spend time in prayer today asking God to help you press on and through the detours. Share your passion with Him and allow His Spirit to ignite that passion to a degree that will keep you going on days that seem like defeat! Write your prayer to the Lord here:

_Lord, thank you for what you have already done in my weight loss journey and thank you for what you will do. Help me to focus on you and not be discouraged when I have detours._

# * Day 3: Compromise is Dangerous

**Reading Assignment:** pp 74-76 in Food, Freedom & Finish Lines!

In Numbers, chapter 32 you can read of when the tribes of Ruben, Gad and the half-tribe of Manasseh decided they wanted to live east of the Jordan River on land they had already conquered. Do you think it was the best of what God wanted them to have? Why or why not?

_No - God had promised them His best - they were settling for "good"_

How often have we rested on our laurels and settled with what we have accomplished thus far. Compromising can be dangerous; keeping us from reaching our promise land. Have you ever settled or compromised concerning a dream you had?

_Yes -_

God's promises are always kept! The Word of God is filled with promises. Until and unless we possess them, they are just words in a book. Look up the word Possess and write its definition.

_to have or own something_

My dictionary defines it as an active verb meaning "to take hold of." The gift of Salvation is offered to anyone who will receive (take hold) and possess it. Your dream, the one God has placed in your heart and filled you with passion for; is yours only if you take hold of it actively and believe God for it. Are you willing to do that and not settle for anything less?

**Food for Thought:** Spend time in God's Word today and claim a promise. Then actively take hold of it and press on through the detours. Refuse to listen to negative thoughts from without or within and keep moving, passionately pursuing your dream.

## * Day 4: Life Change Costs Something

**Reading Assignment:** pp 77-78 in Food, Freedom & Finish Lines!

God wants to do more in us than just change our body shape and size. He wants to do a complete recovery of the whole person...IF we will allow Him to do it! We must get to the place where we trust Him fully for what lies ahead. Are you ready to do that?

_____

_____

_____

Success doesn't happen by accident. God wants us to love Him enough to achieve a healthy goal weight; to live in His fullness, under His protection, and with His provision. On page 78 I wrote about something that must be defeated in order for me to take possession of my new lifestyle. What is it?

_Giants must be defeated_

_____

You too, will have giants in your promise land, and they must be defeated as well. How do we do that? God is certainly able to defeat any giants on our behalf, but we must continue to do our part. In other words, life change costs something. Luke 14:28 says that we should count the cost and make sure we're able to finish.

As you move forward toward your goal, what will it cost you? Maybe it will cost some time to prepare your menus? What about time for consistent exercise? List some of what the costs will be for you to change your lifestyle.

_Time to plan ahead_
_Time for exercise_
_Shopping for and preparing healthy food_

**Food for Thought:** The closer I came to reaching my goal weight, the more difficult it became. Those last 10 pounds seemed impossible but I was determined to finish. Would I make the time? Yes! When I was unable to run, I chose to walk by faith. Will you?

Take time today to write a prayer of commitment to the Lord:

_Lord, I thank you for wanting your very best for me. Help me to do my part to achieve your best and not settle for "good enough." Give me the faith and the perseverance that I need._

## * Day 5: Be an Over comer

**Reading Assignment:** pp 79-80 in Food, Freedom & Finish Lines!

Read 1 John 5:3-5

Challenges are just part of living! The way we look at a challenge will determine how we go about solving it. Think of a recent challenge you've encountered and how you solved it. Then work back and describe how you looked at it when it was encountered.

Were you fearful or did you feel overwhelmed? Or, did you look at it as an opportunity to overcome? The more we face challenges with an over comer's attitude, the sooner we will be able to have the victory we long for. Sometimes we must dig down deep, focus on the goal and take baby steps, one at a time. The worst possible thing we can do is quit! To give up........

The secret to overcoming all obstacles and achieving our goals is to:
_Passionately_
      _Pursue_
            _The Promised Land_

How do I do that, you may ask. Keep your eyes on the goal; chart your progress; exercise discipline; eliminate bad habits and poor excuses. Days when you feel like quitting will seem overwhelming, but if you keep taking the next step...the next right step forward, you will make it.

**Food for Thought:** Ask God to show you your dream. Then obey what He tells you. Establish some short and long term goals. Know that there will be detours and challenges so that when they appear you can ask for help. Above all, don't be afraid to dream.

## * Day 6: Helpful Websites for Success

**Reading Assignment:** Pages 136 -139 Food, Freedom & Finish Lines!

After reviewing the websites I have listed in my book I want to bring some other helpful resources to your attention. These listed below are some websites that may provide you with some tips and guidelines that will help you reach your goals.

**www.firstplace4health.com**
**www.choosemyplate.gov/foodgroups/downloads/myplate/DG2010brochure.pdf**
**www.healthfinder.gov**
**www.letsmove.gov**
**www.eatright.org**

**Food for Thought:** Choose two of the above resources and check them out. Describe whether or not they provided you with help and explain why or why not.

_www.first place 4 health. com - good recipes, like reading_
_success stories_
_www.lets move. gov - good tips_

(Note: if you do not have access to a computer, ask someone to check these resources out for you.)

# * Day 7: Testimonies

**Reading Assignment:** Read testimonies written by Donna Conerly (pp 51-56); Keeli O'Cain (pp 65-69); and Teresa Russell (pp 70-71); then share if you can relate to either of them concerning their struggles on their journey to victory. In what way do you relate?

Donna: _I'm a nurse, too. "We already know this stuff, we just need to do it". Fear because I've lost and gained back before_

Keeli: _perfectionist - have to give up control and surrender daily - Fear of failing_

Teresa: _health problems related to being overweight_

**Food for Thought:** Knowing that others have gone through detours and challenges and have crossed the finish line just as I did, should be an encouragement. We all have similar things going on in our lives and yet we're all different. God knows our hearts and He knows how to get us through any difficulty. It's our job to respond to His leading; obey His commands and trust Him for what we don't understand.
God is faithful all the way to the finish line. Write a prayer today thanking him for his faithfulness.

# Week Four: Barriers

**Word for the Week:**
*But he knows the way that I take; when he has tested me, I will come forth as gold*
Job 23:10 (NIV)

**Weekly Reading Assignment**: Chapters 7-8 in Food, Freedom & Finish Lines!

**Affirmation:** I see each new day as a new and positive adventure. I see problems as exciting challenges that cause me to grow stronger and stronger in my faith.

*"I made it this far because of planning, preparation, and training. And good advice and assistance from others helped me get here too. Experienced marathoners, running books and magazines, life coaches, friends that trained and ran with me, store clerks knowledgeable in training gear have helped me along my way. Can I get past this next barrier?*

## * Day 1: Seeking Advice

**Reading Assignment:** Chapter 7 in Food, Freedom & Finish Lines!

Seeking advice is very important in running a race of importance. When you are running a race toward getting and staying healthy, seeking advice in many areas is vital to success. Which foods, what exercises, how much of this and how few of that…are questions we need answers to

We seek out experts in the field of fitness, nutrition and emotional issues and even spiritual situations. But, there comes a time when we have to sift through the advice and apply what seems to be the correct advice for our individual lives.

All the good advice in the world will not help us succeed if we do not make the necessary changes and get into the race.

Read Joshua 3:5. What did Joshua tell the people they needed to do because the Lord was about to do mighty things?

_consecrate themselves_

Just as the children of Israel stood on the banks of the Jordan River, they had to consecrate themselves and prepare to enter the Promised Land. Are you standing at the banks of your Jordan River right now? Explain

_I need to prepare myself physically, spiritually and emotionally to be successful at weight loss and to be able to enjoy the freedom it will bring_

That place you are at is a faith-building place. God is preparing to do something in you and you can either consecrate yourself and get ready; or turn back. My place at the Jordan River involved my doctor's suggestion to have my excess skin removed. I listened as he asked why I would choose to hang on to it, but could not give him an answer. It was much later through God-arranged circumstances that I finally made the decision to have it removed. Are you hanging on to something that God may be asking you to remove? Think and ponder on that question; pray and then write what is on your heart.

I sought counsel before going through with the surgery…many counsels. Whatever you may be hanging on to, may require counsel before you move into freedom. You may not be facing surgery, but there could be some deeper baggage needing to be unloaded.

Seek out those whom God puts on your heart, both professional and among your friends, pastor, leaders and allow God to give you peace over it.

**Food for Thought:** Removing the excess skin was for me the removal of the final barrier that said, "I'm not going back!"

In a much simpler example, it might be getting rid of all those fat clothes hanging in your closet. God wants to restore you unto Himself. He wants you to be a whole person…mentally, physically, emotionally and spiritually. Let God know how you feel, if you are ready to remove your final barrier to reaching your goal.

_____

_____

_____

_____


## * Day 2: Know Your Options

**Reading Assignment**: pp 89-90 in Food, Freedom & Finish Lines!

After you complete your reading assignment for today, you will understand the daunting process that skin removal surgery was for me. Seeking out wisdom and direction for this procedure caused me to step past my comfort zone.
If we're not willing to step out of our comfort zone, we don't stand much chance of reaching the finish line. You have to know your options…whether it's about skin removal surgery; changing your eating habits; moving; changing careers or any other major life changes! Have you stepped outside your comfort zone recently?
Explain what your options were and how you handled making the decision.

_____

_____

_____


Which of the following areas were you dealing with?

Physical: _____

Mental: _____

Emotional: _____

Spiritual: _____

My surgery allowed me to move into a new freedom from the emotional bondage of food. That final barrier was removed, giving my marriage more strength, and made my faith stronger. You may have more than one area to deal with as well.

What is holding you back?

_____

_____

What about fear? That fear does not come from God. Look up the following Scriptures and write what speaks to you.

Isaiah 41:10 _Don't fear - God is with me and will strengthen and help me._

Psalm 34:4 _If I seek God, He will deliver me from my fears_

**Food for Thought:** Using your concordance, look up other Scriptures regarding fear; then look up those about peace. Write down your thoughts.

_Ps 23    Ps 34:4    1 John 4:18    Ps 27:1_

_Ps 29:11_ _____

_____

## * Day 3: New Strength

**Reading Assignment:** pp 99-100 in Food, Freedom & Finish Lines!

Have you ever made the comment, "I just got my second wind"? You might be working hard physically, exercising; running; cleaning out the garage; or something equally exhausting; and feel as though you simply can't go another step or endure one more minute. Then something occurs and you get a surge of energy and you remark that you got your second wind. It enables you to finish what you started.

I think of it as my new-found strength. Sometimes a runner hears strong encouragement from spectators and other runners, and it gives him/her that new-found strength to finish the course.

Think about a time when you felt you were at the end of your endurance and someone gave you that kind of encouragement. How did you feel? Were you able to keep on going?

_____

_____

_____

Being in a small group like First Place 4 Health has provided me that kind of encouragement. It can come from your prayer partner, the whole group and/or your leader. It works both ways though. You may be the one providing encouragement for someone else so they can get their second wind.

Listen with your heart to your class members when they share. If you feel they need some boosting, don't be shy about giving it. We all need help in this journey.

My new-found strength helped me press forward; giving me renewed energy, self-esteem and confidence. Which of those things might you need right now? Circle all that apply.

Renewed Energy          Self-esteem          Confidence

I discovered that exercise took on a new meaning for me. I love to do many different types of exercise because I have the courage and strength to become the best I can be. And, so can you. I found that if exercise is going to be a part of the rest of my life, and it really has to be, then I need to keep it fun, challenging, exciting and interesting.

**Food for Thought:** How can you be the best you can be? In what areas are you struggling? What would it look like in your life if you were becoming the best you can be physically? Mentally? Emotionally? Spiritually? Think about it and journal what you see.

More energy - able to focus better -
freedom from past hurts
Learning to daily depend on God and use His
strength to be the best that He wants for me

## * Day 4: Changing my Actions

**Reading Assignment:** pp 101-104 in Food, Freedom & Finish Lines!

Changing my actions became my new-found strength. Where do you think real life change happens? Circle one and explain why you chose that particular one.

( In the journey )     at the finish line     because of the finish line

*In the journey is where we learn to depend on God for our strength. We may experience detours, fall down, etc. - but in getting up and getting back of on track we will learn success*

The path to my freedom started when I walked into a FP4H class with the mindset that this was my last hope. Recovery and restoration began in my life that day. I went from unhealthy to strong, from overweight to beauty deeper than my skin.

God's work will continue in the journey all the way to heaven. How about you? As you walk that path to freedom, making changes in your eating and physical lifestyle; do you feel you can believe God for true life changing freedom? Why or why not?

*Yes - He has promised us that. John 8:32 "Then you will know the truth, and the truth will set you free." John 8:36 "If the Son sets you free, you will be free indeed."*

You will notice that each week you have positive affirmations to say aloud daily. For me, they felt like salve applied to a deep, gaping wound. They changed me on the inside. Be sure to write them out and put them where you will see them every day. Speak them aloud and feel the healing they promote. Which of those so far have ministered to you in a positive way to give you hope and strength?

_____

_____

_____

**Food for Thought:** On page 104 I described how the children of Israel traveled toward the Promised Land and laid memorial stones in places where God had shown up to rescue them.

I did the same thing; placing memorial stones to remind me of my life change process. You may want to begin doing it as well. Describe the stones you might place where God has shown up in your life to rescue you.

_____

_____

_____

## * Day 5: Capture the Strength

**Reading Assignment:** pp 105-107 in Food, Freedom & Finish Lines!

This week we have covered a lot of ground, including barriers, freedom and new-found strength. It is important that we realize that God wants His best for us. He wants to knock down those barriers, give us freedom and strength. The very best He has, He wants for us to have. Yet, we too often settle for less than God's very best.

Read Job 23:10
We go through many trials, and hit many barriers on our journey to our Promised Land. What does this verse say will happen after God tries us?

_We will come forth as gold_____

_____

_____

We must not give up! The finish line may be right in front of you. Will you come forth as gold? Only if you do not quit; only if you do not turn back! Some well-meaning people may say, "You look great! Don't take this losing weight too far!"
Let God determine where you cross the finish line. You must not stop until you reach His goals for you, no matter how impossible it may seem.

**Food for Thought:** Marathons are 26.2 miles. It takes a great deal of disciplined training to run or walk a marathon. Accomplishing that feat comes with a huge amount of sacrifice and at times a high personal cost.

What has focusing on your personal race cost you so far?

_____

_____

_____

At the end of a marathon, runners receive a medal to remember the event. It's a physical reward. The reward that God has for those who know Him and win the prize is eternal. So, go for the gold and capture the strength that only God can provide.

## * Day 6: Things to avoid as we Sprint to the Finish Line

**Reading Assignment:** pp 156-157 in Food, Freedom & Finish Lines!

There are three things we must avoid as we head toward the finish line. What are they?

_fear_
_frustration_
_failure_

Read 1 John John 4:18-19 and Romans 8:35 and describe how these two verses replace lies with the truth of God's Word, and avoid being fearful.

_Nothing can separate us from God's love_
_There is no fear in love - perfect love drives out fear_
_We love because He first loved us._

Read Galatians 6:9. How does this verse help you avoid frustration along your journey?

_Reassurance that I will succeed if I don't give up_

_____

_____

Read 1 Corinthians 15:57-58. What does this verse instruct you to do to avoid failure?

_Stand firm. Let nothing move me. Always give_
_myself fully to the work of the Lord_

_____

Write out 2 Timothy 4:7 in the space provided below. Now write it out on an index card and memorize it. Post it in places to remind you not to give up.

*I have fought the good fight, I have finished the race, I have kept the faith.*

## * Day 7: Memorial Stones

**Reading Assignment**: Review your reading assignments from this week in Food, Freedom and Finish lines!

This week you read about how I used memorial stones to mark the places in my life where God showed up and rescued me. Today, take a nature walk; (maybe in your own back yard), and find appropriate stones that you can use to make your own memorial.

What will your memorial look like? I am not sure but it should represent the places in your life concerning your weight loss journey where God showed up.

The number of stones is up to you depending on where and how often God rescued you. Be prepared to share with your class in your next meeting.

**<u>Food for Thought</u>**: Write down the stones you find and the names you are giving them and why?

_____

_____

_____

_____

_____

# Week Five: Ongoing Power

**Word for the Week:** *"You have persevered and have endured hardships for my name, and have not grown weary."* Revelation 2:3

**Weekly Reading Assignment:** Chapters 9-10 in Food, Freedom & Finish Lines!

**Affirmation:** I am sustained by the love of Christ.

*As I draw near the finish, my body is tired and my muscles ache, my feet are tired and heavy. Not much farther now. As I draw closer, others pass me. I push harder. I tell myself, "I can do it. I'm almost there."*

Sometimes the closer we get to reaching our goal, the more difficult it seems. It doesn't matter if you're 10 pounds away from your healthy weight goal or 10 pounds away from moving down to the next plateau. We think that our race would get easier by now, but instead, it seems more difficult.

This is where we learn to apply that patience and obedience we've learned about along the way. It's where we find out if the life change is for real.

## * Day 1: My Nathan

**Reading Assignment:** pp 109-110 in Food, Freedom & Finish Lines!

Remember the Prophet, Nathan (2 Samuel 12)? As a Prophet, his job was to confront sin...even if it was sin of a king. It must have taken a lot of courage to speak to David and make him realize that what he did was wrong. So Nathan told David a story about two men in a town, one rich and one poor. Read 2 Samuel 12 and in your own words describe what happened and how David reacted when he realized he was the villain in Nathan's story.

The rich man took the only lamb the poor man had & killed it to feed a traveler. At first David was angry - he told Nathan the rich man should die. When Nathan told David it was him, David confessed his sin and accepted the Lord's discipline.

Have you ever had someone confront you in this way (or have you had to confront someone else like this)? If so, describe the situation and how you (or they), responded.

_____

_____

_____

My Nathan helped me to realize I needed the right kind of reinforcement, in the form of a nutritionist. Seeking this kind of help was, for me, a sign of willingness to reach deep for the right answers. I needed qualified counsel. The best thing she did for me was to challenge me to take the principles I'd learned in FP4H to a new level.

Read the second paragraph on page 112. What was my first thought?
_rebellion_
What did the Lord remind me of and say to me?
Her declaration of surrender to Him & to patiently wait on Him. God was showing her the way & told her to walk in obedience & trust Him.

Whatever your goal is; wherever you are on your journey to your Promised Land, be sure, you will need reminding of the declarations you have made to God. And God is faithful, He will remind you!

God may be telling you:
*"I am showing you the way."*
*"Walk in obedience."*
*"Trust me in this."*

God may want to bring in new people to hold you to a higher level of accountability…a Nathan who is not afraid to speak truth to you. Recognize it when it happens and thank God for it.

**Food for Thought:** Do you have a Nathan in your life; someone courageous enough to tell you the truth and help direct you where God wants you to go? Pray that God will send a Nathan to you to help you as you journey to your Promised Land; regardless of how far away you are; and that you will be open to hearing the truth and acting upon it.

# * Day 2: Helping Others

**Reading Assignment:** pp 113-114 in Food, Freedom & Finish Lines!

As weight begins to come off and the numbers on the scale go down, we become more determined and committed to make good choices and follow the plan. It matters to us. But, God does something in that whole process; He begins to create in us a desire to help others learn what He's been teaching us. Who do you know that would benefit from being in this program and journeying with you?

_____

_____

_____

When I attended the FP4H Summit in Houston, TX, I was asked to give my testimony. As a result, I challenged others there to go to the finish line with me. Many stepped out in faith and I went home with a new budding hope. My accountability team expanded.

There are many hurting people in the world, desperate for an answer, looking for a way out of the isolation that often comes as a result of obesity. How do we help them? By way of our testimony! When we stand before someone healed of our own obesity and give God the glory; guess what? The Holy Spirit will carry the message to intended hearts, convicting and encouraging them to join us.

Today is a good day to begin forming your testimony. You may not yet be at your goal, but you still can testify as to how God is moving you closer and closer each day. Think right now of how far you have come since you've been in FP4H, and write down how God brought you to this place. What have you learned that would benefit others?

_When I depend on God's strength I can resist_
_temptation. With determination, I am finding_
_success and I am thankful. Focusing on_
_Bible study is helping me grow closer to God_

We truly need each other. You may be halfway to your goal while someone else is just beginning their journey. Someone else may be at their goal and they will encourage you as you continue your journey. The truth is, we must find our own pace and run the race that God has for us individually. You can't run mine and I can't run yours.

Who do you know that needs encouragement right now? Who do you know that you can ask for encouragement from?

_____

_____

_____

**Food for Thought:** The Promised Land is there for you to claim. Gather others to come along and join you as each of you journey toward your own Promised Land. Your experiences and setbacks might help them; just as theirs can assist you over difficult days.
Pray about enlarging your accountability group by sharing your testimony with others. What can you say; who will you say it to?

_____

_____

_____

## * Day 3: Tough Times

**Reading Assignment:** pp 116-117 in Food, Freedom & Finish Lines!

When things are going well, we must not relax our guard. I was doing great but still not at my goal, so I was determined and committed to walk in obedience.
By teaching FP4H I was held accountable in my Bible study, Scripture memorization and of course, weigh-ins. I ran a half marathon and my friends surprised me with a victory/birthday party (minus the cake). I was so close to my goal.
I was about to enter the two toughest months of the year…yes, the holidays of Thanksgiving and Christmas and cold weather.
Signing up for another half marathon in January must have been done when I was delirious, but there it was. I had to train and reevaluate my food and exercise plans, and set the pace for the finish.

Could I finish and get to goal this time? Then the realization set in that "Freedom cost something." If I was to finish strong, I had to be willing to pay the price that success required. I knew I couldn't do it…I didn't have it in me…But Christ could and He did!

Read 2 Corinthians 4:7 and write it out.

_But we have this treasure in jars of clay to show that this all-surpassing power is from God and not from us._

My being weak is where God steps in and takes control, infusing His power into me. The same power that raised Christ from the dead, that same power is in me. Power to finish strong! I could not cross that finish line and claim victory unless I acknowledged that it was His divine power that carried me.

So there I was, this earthen vessel; trusting in God to carry me to victory. Of course, with holiday time around the corner, the devil whispers, "What if the scales don't move? What if you don't make goal?" My efforts alone won't make it happen.
I have freedom to choose to eat well, exercise and trust God. Then God asked, "Will you go back? Will you stop being obedient?" If I don't succeed in reaching my goal, will I go back to bondage of food, and say that God couldn't fulfill His promise? NO!

What about you? When holidays approach or tough times appear on the scene, what will you do? Will you continue to trust God or will you go back to Egypt? Think about it......

---

---

**Food for Thought:** Do you have a plan for when holidays come around (they do each year, you know)? Are you determined and committed and in till the finish? As you make your plans to handle those times, remember that God wants to carry you across that finish line. Your plan must include walking in obedience and trusting the Lord every step of the way. Are you ready?

---

---

## * Day 4: Celebrate

**Reading Assignment:** Read the personal reflection on page 117 in Food, Freedom & Finish Lines!

Celebrations are fun and we all enjoy celebrating both small and large victories. From losing 1 pound, getting off sugar, planning a week's worth of meals, to reaching a goal; we can always find something to celebrate. What have you celebrated since you began this journey?

_____

_____

_____

I had two best friends during this part of my journey, what were they?

_patience_
_consistent obedience_

Regarding patience, I had to learn to be patient with myself, others and the Lord.
Regarding Obedience, I had to learn to surrender daily to the work that He was doing in me; and especially to put it into practice as I learned.

Who might your two best friends be during your journey, and what must you learn from them?

_patience - wt loss won't be quick - Don't quit!_
_daily surrender - I need the Lord's help and_
_guidance every day!_

Like writing a novel: you haven't written one until you finish it. You must be willing to put in the time and effort to finishing. In actuality, finishing is just the beginning of the journey. We learn through the process of finishing how to continue to choose well daily.
Do you want to celebrate success and finish? Then you have to be willing to pay the price that success requires. Your life change process, like mine, has to be a priority for you, regardless of what it costs.

**Food for Thought:** What will your celebration look like? Do you have a picture in your mind of finishing your race by reaching your goal? Who will you credit for your success? Who will you tell? Can you see it? Spend time today visualizing the day of your success; the day when you step on the scale and it smiles back with your perfect number. How will you feel and celebrate?

_____

_____

_____


## * Day 5: Making Goal

**Reading Assignment:** pp 119-122 in Food, Freedom & Finish Lines!

_Then I see it. Penned in large letters, hanging above the street, the word I have longed to see – FINISH. With my arms raised high in triumph, I cross the finish line!_

I thanked God that day for the ability to finish, for through Him alone, all things are possible. I stepped on the scales and saw 147 pounds…my goal weight! My BMI dropped to the normal range, as did my body fat. It had been a long journey. The last 10 pounds were by far the hardest to lose. Turn to Isaiah 40:31(KJV) and meditate on it a few minutes, then read it over again. Fill in the blanks.

But they that **wait** upon the **Lord** shall **renew** their **strength** ; they shall mount up with **wings** as eagles; they shall **run**, and not be **fai** ; and they shall _____, and not _____

The first blank you filled in is "wait," and whom do you wait upon?

_____

When you wait upon the Lord you will be able to take off and fly like an eagle, effortlessly! That is freedom dear friend, freedom from the bondage that food has on you. I have finally found freedom; I am still in the race and plan to bring others with me. I may be at my goal but there are others I want to help get here. It's time to build a heritage of lasting life change.

How do you view FP4H? Circle all that apply.

\*A diet \*Weight loss program \*A wellness program that changes lives

Are you in this with the Lord or merely using it to shed a few pounds? My friend, what you learn through FP4H is that the Lord wants to help you be transformed in all four areas of your life; not just in the physical. He wants to use you as a channel of blessing in the lives of others struggling in their journey. My prayer is that you are in it with Him and will wait upon the Lord so that you too may experience the freedom He has for you.

**Food for Thought:** Think about ways in which God may use you this week to spread the word about how God can help people through FP4H. Perhaps God is speaking to you about starting a new FP4H group. If so, don't tune Him out, but ask Him to show you what you should do next.

Use this time to journal about what you feel God is saying to you right now.

*Praying that God will make it clear to me if I should start a group and if so, when (this fall or after I've completed another session) and am closer to goal weight)*

**\* Day 6: Exercise Tips**

**Reading Assignment:** pp 164-168 in Food, Freedom & Finish Lines!

The most important tip regarding exercise is that you must start! We can build on that and move to different levels. Another tip is to stop saying I "have to" exercise. Begin now to start saying, I "get to" exercise.

You deserve it. Think of it as a pampering you do for yourself to make your body more efficient. When you get a massage, think of all the benefits you get from that massage and jot down a few.

Massages are very beneficial to our physical bodies; they rid our bodies of toxins, increase blood flow, and work our muscles. Massages are also beneficial to our mental balance.

Now compare that with exercise and jot down some benefits, only this time, add additional ones that come just from exercise.

_Strengthens muscles, burns calories,_
_relieves stress, increases metabolism, burns fat_

Exercise has many more benefits and is not just a feel good pampering. You "Get To" exercise and bring your body health benefits that will increase your ability to do all you need to do and to serve God as long as possible.

Today on pages 164-167, read through the eight tips.

Are there any of those tips that you have already implemented into your new healthy lifestyle? If so which ones?

_doing @ least 5-10 min/day_
_garmin step tracker / music_

Now select two that you feel you need to work on implementing into your life. Which two will you select and why?

_Mix it up (to keep motivated)_
_get walking partner_

Food for Thought: Ask yourself, "How do I feel about exercise?" Do you look forward to it, dread it or simply endure it? Remember, you "get to" exercise! This is something nice that you get to do in order to get yourself healthy and strong physically. Perhaps you may need to talk to God about your attitude towards exercise. Spend time today with Him and write out how you feel afterwards.

# * Day 7: Your Testimony

**Read Assignment:** Review back over the reading assignments from this week

Today, you will begin forming your testimony and hopefully be prepared to share it with your class at the end of this session. Think of your testimony in three parts: where you were (health-wise); How God worked in and through you during this session; and how you plan to use what you have learned in FP4H to make this a life change and help others find success.

Let's look at the first part: Where were you physically with your health/weight before joining FP4H? Describe your weight, general health, any diseases (diabetes, high blood pressure, high cholesterol, etc.). Also, where were you spiritually in your walk with the Lord; where were you emotionally and mentally? A few sentences in each are fine for now. You will expand it over time.

_Weight was at all-time high, ↑ BP, ↑ cholesterol, fatigue. I had started daily Bible reading/quiet time but felt my weight was the one area of my life I could not "conquer" - felt defeated, depressed._

Next, write out specifically how God changed you during this session. Maybe he has worked on your attitude? How about eating habits? Maybe it has been your memory? Could it be in your relationships?

_God has given me hope/renewed determination through FP4H. I have a more positive attitude and healthier eating habits._

Lastly, what do you plan to do with what you've learned through FP4H? Will you give your testimony? Start a FP4H group? What is the Lord calling you to do? Be specific.

_I want to work on my testimony & possibly start a FP4H group at my church_

**Food For Thought:** My book, "Food, Freedom & Finish Lines" is my testimony concerning my journey to my Promised Land. I don't expect you to write a book (unless God directs you to), but putting onto paper how God has/is working to transform your life is very important.

# Week Six: Memorial Stones

**Word for the Week:**
Joshua 4:22 *"Israel crossed the Jordan on dry ground. For the Lord your God dried up the Jordan before you until you had crossed over."*

**Weekly Reading Assignment:** Chapter 11 in Food, Freedom & Finish Lines!

**Affirmation:** God always causes me to triumph in Christ.

This week is our final week of study, but I believe one of the most important weeks in our study. Everything you have learned thus far I pray you have made active in your life and are well on your way to your own finish line to enter your Promised Land.

I wonder how you will use that wisdom to build a heritage of life change. I will be sharing with you, my memorial stones which are a reminder to me and to others that a life of freedom is truly possible and reachable. You may be thinking, "How does this happen?" Let's begin by looking at my memorial stones.

## * Day 1: The Stone of Truth

**Reading Assignment:** pages 124 and half of 125 in Food, Freedom & Finish Lines!

The Stone of Truth is the _____ stone. Life change begins with truth. Read Psalm 25:12-14. Fearing God means recognizing God is holy, almighty, righteous, pure, all-knowing, all-powerful, and all wise. God is truth and my life change began when I recognized that humble respect and reverence is due Him. Life change is not possible without Him.

How do you view God?

_____

_____

_____

I came to see myself as weak, sinful, frail, and desperately needy. I am unable to make the right decisions or choices daily on my own. I know I need God as my Stone of Truth! How do you see yourself?

_____

_____

_____

God's power and strength can break the chains of bondage. Food does not have to remain a powerful stronghold in your life. When you view God as Truth and almighty powerful; and see yourself as weak and needy; God can/will help you find freedom.
Please understand we all have the ability to lose some weight on our own but we will never find true freedom without the power of Christ.

**Food for Thought**: This memorial stone, The Stone of Truth, also reminds me that I will never go back. Think about finding a stone to help you remember to walk in faith and obedience with an all-powerful God to lead you safely across that river to your Promised Land. Write a scripture on it and place it in a place of importance so you can constantly be reminded of this truth.

## * Day 2: The Stone of Surrender

**Reading Assignment**: pp 125-126 in Food, Freedom & Finish Lines!

My second stone is The Stone of Surrender. I chose to surrender my mind and body to the truth that has set me free. What do you think happens when you do that?

_____

_____

_____

When I chose to surrender my mind and body to the truth, I began to think differently about food and exercise. I didn't see things the same way. Sure, I love to eat; don't we all? I don't eat food I don't like.

The thing that happened to me when I surrendered my mind and body willingly to the truth was that food no longer held a place of power! I now choose the healthiest thing possible and have a deep desire to honor the Lord with my body instead of heaping abuse on it from poor food choices.

Some days I choose poorly. I enjoy ice cream, and have learned how to make it part of my plan; but there is no guilt or condemnation for enjoying ice cream because it IS part of the plan.

Exercise is another area that required surrender. I can easily talk myself out of going to the gym, but my accountability group keeps me from faltering. Most days I love going and I'm thankful for them. When I don't feel like going I'm thankful for a team who will not allow me to quit.
Every choice to surrender makes the next choice easier. The key here is surrender. What do you need to surrender today so that you can mark it with a Stone of Surrender?

_____

_____

_____


**Food for Thought:** Every day offers us a new opportunity to surrender to the truth that will set us free. Day by day, one step at a time, our desires will change as we willingly surrender things to the Lord. He desires for you to be healthy and when we do that, we honor Him with our body; the body He created.
Today, surrender an area that keeps food in power. Watch what God will do!


## * Day 3: The Stone of Obedience

**Reading Assignment:** pp 127-128 in Food, Freedom & Finish Lines!

Okay, don't stop here and tune me out. That word Obedience can do that sometimes. Another stone is the Stone of Obedience and it is at the top of my memorial for a reason.

None of the other stones will be useful or powerful without The Stone of Obedience. Is there an area of your life where you are not being obedient to what you know God wants you to do?

_____

_____

_____

Even today I continue to practice the components of life change I have written about and you have learned about throughout my book, Food, Freedom & Finish Lines! The act of obedience ensures that I do…on the days I feel like it and on the days I don't feel like it.

Review the chapters you have been through in this study and find the components of life change that have helped you the most. Reflect on and describe how they have helped you.

_____

_____

_____

My memorial is in place; Three large stones. Name them:

_____

_____

_____

What will your memorial look like?

_____

_____

_____

**Food for Thought:** Think about the memorial you will make. Use time today to maybe go out and select three large stones. You actually may have more stones. It is between you and God so allow God to show you. Choose those stones that mark specific things God has instilled in you through this program.

# * Day 4: What's Next?

**Reading Assignment**: pages 127-129 in Food, Freedom & Finish Lines!

There are two elements I have identified to long-term life change success. Today I'll share my first new goal. It is to live life fully. What do I mean by that? In your own words describe what I mean after reading the bottom of page 127 that starts out, "My first new goal."

_____

_____

_____

When our roots go down deep in the Promised Land, we can weather the storms without giving up our new way of life. The key here is that our roots must go down deep. We learn the basics when we first begin, but we must go deeper.

We learn the food plan well and begin planning and implementing new foods, but we must go deeper. We incorporate an exercise plan into our daily life, but we must go deeper.
Deeper with the Lord! We must allow Him to transform our mind, our thinking. We don't want to revert back to the old ways. Think about how you thought when you began this program. Has your thinking changed regarding food and exercise? In what ways?

_____

_____

_____

Read the section on page 127 about the afternoon I walked on the beach. Then list some of the things in your life that affect the big picture.

_____

_____

_____

Now look at the little grains of stress I mentioned and describe what they can lead to.

_____

_____

**Food for Thought:** When those little grains of sand change the big picture, our life change deteriorates into the same old habits. Decide now how you will identify and address stress in order to be successful and really live your life fully.

_____

_____

_____


## * Day 5: My Next New Goal

**Reading Assignment:** the remainder of page 128 through 130 in Food, Freedom & Finish Lines!

What's next involves living my life fully, but it also includes helping others. My desire, as I find my way in the land of maintenance, practicing life change and moving from amateur to professional is to make a difference in the lives of others. Why? So that the heritage I pass on will be one of hope, help and healing. To do this I must continue to set goals for myself and encourage others like you. I want to see others become healthy and healed.

Right where you are now, what kind of goals have you set for yourself in each of the four areas of your life?

Physical:_____

_____

Mental:_____

_____

Emotional:_____

_____

Spiritual:_____

_____

Are these fresh goals or are they the same ones you set back when you started? Have you reached any of them yet?

_____

_____

_____

If I am to help others find their way into life change, I must constantly re-evaluate my goals and be sure that I'm not stagnant. If I'm not reaching previous goals, perhaps they need to be adjusted.
Today, spend some time looking at your goals and see if yours may need adjusting. Write out your new ones or the adjusted old ones.

_____

_____

_____

**Food for Thought**: I started at 339 pounds and finished at 147 pounds; a long journey indeed. Sometimes I look in the mirror and expect to see that other 192 pounds. As I continue to walk in obedience I pray the Lord will remove all traces of that image from my mind.

Do you have an image in your mind you would like the Lord to remove? Describe it and then spend time in prayer and perhaps journal your prayer. He's waiting to hear from you.

_____

_____

_____

## * Day 6: Mindset and Expectations

**Reading Assignment:** Review and reflect back on page 129 through 131 in Food, Freedom and Finish Lines!

Yesterday I shared on page 129 that I had the wrong mindset and expectation. Races are hard because they are supposed to be a measure of endurance and hard work. I don't know where I got the idea that race day would be easy but that was my mindset.

My expectation was that I would breeze through it all. Have you ever gone into something with that kind of thinking? Maybe when you started FP4H?

_____

_____

_____

The race we are in through this weight loss thing, is hard work; a measure of endurance. There are some hills that will test us and leave us wondering how we could have ever thought it would be a breeze. But, that day of my race as I plowed up the hill at Lefluer's Bluff in the middle of the race, I wondered how often in my life I had the same idea about God's blessings.

Running on empty and feeling tired, I hung my head. I wanted to quit. When I looked up, there they were; my husband and my best friends, running alongside me, encouraging me, and telling me I was doing great. Tears flowed down my face and in that moment I knew I could finish. God went through it with me all the way, but He sent reinforcements.

My goal now, with my new mindset and expectations, is to cheer, urge and encourage you and others to make life changes that matters. Life Change that is real and lasting! Will you join me?

_____

_____

## * Day 7: Victory and Freedom

Reading Assignment: read 2 Timothy 4:7

You made it through this study! Today is not the end, but the beginning. Where you go next and how you use what you've learned, will determine your life change. Tomorrow is where your victory and freedom begin. Step into it and claim your race. You may or may not be at your goal. That might take six weeks, months or years. But tomorrow is the first day of your victory and freedom from the bondage of food.

The race is not easy but you have persevered. How do you feel having completed this study?

_____

_____

_____

What is the next step you feel the Lord wants you to take?

_____

_____

_____

What is the most important thing you feel you have learned while completing this study?

_____

_____

_____

I keep pictures of the old me as part of my memorial, of where I have come from and where I am determined never to return. I urge you to spend time today gathering your memorial things and dedicate them to God. It is important to share with your class members, how you feel and where you are headed. Be honest and open with your group.

Do you still have hills to climb? Still have stubborn pounds to lose? Share your feelings of how you plan to conquer the hills and chisel off those pounds. Write a couple paragraphs based on how you plan to move closer to and cross that finish line.

I encourage you also to write to me (**Glenna@netdoor.com**) and let me become one of your encouragers in this journey.

Remember don't quit and don't give up! Your finish line is just ahead. I will see you at the finish!

Change Your Mind! Change Your Body! Change Your Life!

Faithfully His,

_Joyce_

## About the Author

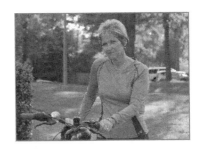

**Joyce Ainsworth** has been a lifetime resident of Mississippi, a dedicated wife to husband Glenn and mother to their five children; now grown. Through FP4H, she has been successful at losing and maintaining a weight loss of 192 pounds. Joyce speaks at seminars, conferences, and other events throughout the country. She coordinates the FP4H Ministry for her home church and teaches FP4H classes. She also serves as Regional Director for FP4H for the Southern States of the United States.

Joyce is a successful business owner and as a writer and motivational speaker; she shares her experiences, offers insight, and is committed to helping others find hope, help, and healing out of the bondage to food and other addictions. Joyce is a ISSA Certified Specialist in Fitness Nutrition and also conducts cooking demonstrations and workshops on healthy living for a better life.

**"Freedom is not a program," she says, "It is a lifestyle."**

**Her Motto:**
**Change Your Mind~ Change Your Body~ Change your Life!**

# Invite Joyce Ainsworth to speak at your next event

Contact her for a list of speaking topics
Email: glenna@netdoor.com
www.joyceainsworth.com

Read Joyce's weekly blog
mondaymovationsbyjoyce

## Connect with Joyce

 Facebook – Joyce Ainsworth

@joyceainsworth

Read more about Joyce at:
http://www.firstplace4health.com/stories/34/joyce_ainsworth

Joyce's new cookbook is now available:
## *Simply Healthy Recipes ~ Food for the Body and Soul*
*Taste and See How "Good" healthy can be!*

*New Book Now Available*
## *Nutrition for Life*
## *Food and Fitness Tips for Success*

Order your copy today at www.joyceainsworth.com
or at glenna@netdoor.com
Copies are also available on Amazon.com

Made in the USA
San Bernardino, CA
10 May 2015